SUPER CHARGE WITH SUPER FOODS

- FIGHT DISEASE
- BOOST YOUR IMMUNITY
- REVERSE THE AGING PROCESS
- AND IMPROVE VITALITY!

DELIA QUIGLEY AND B.E. HORTON, MS, RD

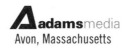

Avon, Massachusetts

Published by Adams Media,
a division of F+W Media, Inc.
57 Littlefield Street, Avon, MA 02322. U.S.A.

Contains material adapted and abridged from *The Everything® Superfoods Book*,
by Delia Quigley, CNC with Brierley E. Wright, MS, RD, copyright © 2008
by F+W Media, Inc., ISBN 10: 1-59869-682-3, ISBN 13: 978-1-59869-682-0.

ISBN 10: 1-4405-0236-6
ISBN 13: 978-1-4405-0236-1
eISBN 10: 1-4405-0709-0
eISBN 13: 978-1-4405-0709-0

Printed in the United States of America.

10 9 8 7 6 5 4 3 2 1

Library of Congress Cataloging-in-Publication Data
is available from the publisher.

This publication is designed to provide accurate and authoritative information with regard to the subject matter covered. It is sold with the understanding that the publisher is not engaged in rendering legal, accounting, or other professional advice. If legal advice or other expert assistance is required, the services of a competent professional person should be sought.

—From a *Declarations of Principles* jointly adopted by a Committee of the American Bar Association and a Committee of Publishers and Associations

Many of the designations used by manufacturers and sellers to distinguish their product are claimed as trademarks. Where those designations appear in this book and Adams Media was aware of a trademark claim, the designations have been printed with initial capital letters.

This book is available at quantity discounts for bulk purchases.
For information, please call 1-800-289-0963.

CONTENTS

TOP TEN REASONS FOR EATING SUPERFOODS

1. Each Superfood listed contributes significant vitamins, minerals, and other nutrients to support the proper functions of your body.
2. Numerous international scientific studies confirm that Superfoods should be a part of your diet on a daily and weekly basis.
3. The vitamins and minerals contained in Superfoods are more easily absorbed and assimilated by the body than any supplements.
4. The twenty-five Superfoods listed are natural whole foods that have helped human beings evolve on this planet over thousands and thousands of years.
5. The high amounts of antioxidants in Superfoods protect your body from damage caused by free radicals in the environment.
6. Superfoods can be eaten for everyday nutritional support and can be used to help cleanse, heal, and rejuvenate the body.
7. People who eat Superfoods harvested from the sea have been shown to have fewer problems from mineral depletion and tend to live longer, healthier lives.
8. The Superfood garlic has been called the natural antibiotic for its powerful antibacterial, antifungal, and antiviral properties.
9. Superfoods provide essential carbohydrates, proteins, and quality fats needed in your daily diet.
10. All the Superfoods have been recommended by the U.S. Dietary Guidelines for achieving and maintaining optimal health.

INTRODUCTION

SUPERCHARGE YOUR HEALTH, LIFE, AND HAPPINESS

No doubt you've read about the high rates of obesity, heart disease, and cancer affecting not only adults but young children and teenagers as well. What you eat affects the state of your health. Approximately 1.6 million out of a total 2.1 million deaths a year in the United States are related to poor nutrition, according to the former Surgeon General C. Everett Koop. This can be easily remedied by eating a well-balanced diet of whole grains, fruit, vegetables, beans, legumes, nuts, seeds, and lean animal protein—and eliminating junk-food snacks. If you're looking to change what you eat, then you probably already know that the difficult part is taking those first few steps toward doing something about it. It's easy to feel trapped in an endless loop of cravings, weight gain, and depression. Perhaps you've lost a few pounds trying the latest fad diet only to regain twice as much as you lost, leaving you feeling frustrated and defeated.

Well, if you've picked up this book you've taken your first step toward changing your health and life for the better. If you were to replace just one of the less healthy foods you eat each day with one of the Superfoods listed in this book, you would be taking twenty-five steps toward significantly improving your diet. Think about it: By reading one chapter at a time and implementing the knowledge you gain, you can successfully cleanse, purify, renew, rejuvenate, and rebuild your body. That is the power of eating a Superfoods diet. What's more, an overwhelming evidence of research points to the benefits of eating specific whole foods for optimal health and well-being.

As a wise and ancient philosopher once wrote, "The journey of a thousand miles begins with the first step." This book gives you the first twenty-five steps—from broccoli preventing cancer to salmon boosting your mood and beans being budget friendly—to supercharge your health, life, and happiness. The remainder of this chapter will introduce each of the twenty-five Superfoods, all of which will help you sustain a healthy life. Let's begin!

WHAT ARE SUPERFOODS?

Superfoods are particular types of food containing high amounts of phyto-nutrients (or phytochemicals), organic components of plants that promote health. In fact, you're probably familiar with some of the more common ones: carotenoids, polyphenols, isoflavones, etc. Phytochemicals are not essential for life in the way that other vitamins and minerals are. Individually, phytochemicals offer specific important health benefits, and taken as a whole they boast a major defense against disease and the ravages of free radicals, environmental toxins, and heavy-metal contamination. You can find numerous articles on the benefits of foods considered "super," but for the most part the twenty-five foods detailed in this book can almost unanimously be found on all the Superfood lists.

THE FAMILIAR AND NOT-SO-FAMILIAR

The majority of these Superfoods should not appear unusual; as a matter of fact, you probably eat most if not all of them on a daily basis. Take apples for instance, a favorite snack loaded with antioxidants that can be eaten plain or with a smear of nut butter or transformed into an apple crumb pie. Blueberries, on any list of favorites, are low in fat and high in fiber and easy to use in smoothies or smothered in another Superfood—probiotic-rich yogurt. Perfect for your digestive system, a plain, tart yogurt can be puréed with the powerful cruciferous supervegetable broccoli for a healthy soup or vegetable dip. Quinoa may be new to most of you, coming only recently from the mountains of Peru, but its high protein content makes it a must-have on your shopping list. And it pairs well with chopped almonds. Not many people can live without their chocolate—the darker the healthier, so go ahead and find out why you can enjoy a bite of decadence—or eggs for breakfast. Add half of a vitamin C-rich grapefruit for a double dose of Superfoods at breakfast.

This Superfoods list would not be complete without both land and sea vegetables. The oceans provide an amazing storehouse of mineral-rich foods to rival the most nutrient-dense land produce: dulse, arame, hijiki, and kombu are proving themselves to be effective in weight-loss studies and preventing osteoporosis.

South of the border they know how to appreciate the healthy fats in avocado. These are the "good" fats you want to include in your diet because when you balance them with a few sprigs of the blood-cleansing parsley, everything flows along nicely. Add wild salmon to the menu and you have the ideal source of omega-3 fatty acids, essential fats your body needs for clear beautiful skin, shiny hair, and a well-functioning brain. Beans, a budget-friendly vegetarian source of protein, provide you with nutrients and fiber, and there is a wide variety to choose from. Kale and cabbage are powerful cancer-fighting vegetables that are super easy to prepare.

Meanwhile, you can sip your antioxidants in green tea, get a good night's sleep with sour cherries, and support your prostate and bones with a handful of pumpkin seeds for a snack. You can always add the tea and seeds to a blender with mineral-rich chlorella, spirulina, blue-green algae, or wheat-grass juice, some frozen blueberries, and sweetener of choice for a quick and healthy smoothie.

Wondering what to eat for breakfast? Look no further than a bowl of the mother of all grains—whole oats cooked overnight in the Crock-Pot and served warm the next morning with a few tablespoons of walnuts or almonds. For lunch, a powerhouse salad of cooked sweet potatoes—high in vitamin A—and cooked kale topped with toasted walnuts and tossed with an apple-cider vinaigrette allows for easy digestion and assimilation of nutrients.

THE NUTRITION AND SCIENCE OF SUPERFOODS

The understanding of our nutritional needs based on the quality of food intake has been a sometimes slow scientific process, but one from which we are constantly and continuously learning. When fast foods were first introduced to the American public, they were thought to be an antidote to our increasingly busy lifestyles. Now you see the detrimental results of this way of thinking. Along with a convenient diet came a fair amount of processed food and a host of other unhealthy habits: Serving sizes increased while at the same time people became less active. More refined carbohydrates were consumed with higher amounts of hydrogenated oils used to prepare them. The intake of omega-3 fatty acids declined, as refined-sugar and omega-6 fatty acids consumption increased. Fruits and vegetables became a small side dish and high-fat dairy products such as cheese and ice cream were consumed in overabundance. American diets became more refined and processed. And at the same time Americans ate fewer varieties of foods. Studies show that Americans typically rotate ten meals over and over in the course of a week. Does this sound like you? If so, chances are your body is missing out on some of the necessary nutrients needed to sustain health.

Today scientific research shows repeatedly that eating a balanced whole-foods diet, made up of a variety of foods including the twenty-five Superfoods, will lower rates and reduce Americans' risk of obesity, diabetes, heart disease, and cancer. So, go ahead and rotate ten meals a week—just make them with the foods on the Superfoods list.

EATING FOR OPTIMAL HEALTH

Most foods contain a combination of two groups that you will want to include when planning your food menu: macronutrients, so called because the body needs more of them; and micronutrients, nutrients required in only small amounts—these include vitamins and minerals.

Macronutrients include carbohydrates, fats, and proteins, which are the foods your body uses for energy and growth.

- ▶ **Carbohydrates include all starches and sugars and are the body's main source of energy.** Each gram of carbohydrate provides 4 calories. Most foods contain carbohydrates.
- ▶ **Fats pack a lot of energy.** Each gram of fat provides 9 calories. There are three kinds of fat: saturated, monounsaturated, and polyunsaturated. Animal fats, coconut oils, and dairy fats, which remain solid at room temperature, are saturated fats, sometimes referred to as unhealthy fats. Unsaturated fats include vegetable fat and oils; they remain liquid at room temperature and are usually referred to as healthy fats.

► **Protein, like carbohydrates, provides energy at 4 calories per gram.** They are the body's building materials: muscle, skin, bone, and hair are made up largely of proteins. In addition, every cell contains proteins called enzymes, which facilitate chemical reactions in the body; cells could not function without these enzymes. The body uses proteins to make antibodies, or disease-fighting chemicals, and certain hormones such as insulin, which serve as chemical messengers in the body. (Other hormones, such as the female hormone estrogen, are not made from proteins.) Meat, poultry, fish, dairy products, eggs, cereals, legumes, and nuts are all good sources of protein.

A well-balanced meal includes each of the macronutrients, so try to include each of them in your menu plans.

THE USDA FOOD PYRAMID

The USDA has created a food pyramid (*www.mypyramid.gov*) as a guide for balancing your diet with proper foods. They also offer personalized eating plans—based on your recommended calorie intake—to help you plan and asses your food choices. To balance your daily intake of food, you'll need to eat a calorie range of no less than 1,200 calories made up of 20–25 percent protein, 50–55 percent carbohydrates (with the emphasis on vegetables, fruits, and whole grains), and 20–30 percent good/healthy fats. The USDA food pyramid is a good place to begin putting together some sample menus and create a full day of meals, snacks, and drinks. At first it may seem a bit overwhelming as you learn how many grams of protein, carbohydrates, and fats you and your family need, but little by little it will all come together for you. Here's an example, based on 2,000 calories a day: 6 ounces of whole grains; 2½ cups of vegetables; 2 cups of fruit; 3 cups of milk products; 5½ ounces animal protein and beans; 6 teaspoons of quality oil; and 267 discretionary calories.

To break it down further, your day could look like this:

- ▶ 5–7 servings of whole grains = 1 slice of bread, ½ cup of cereal, ½ cup of whole grains, ½ cup of pasta, 1 tortilla
- ▶ 3–5 servings of fruit = 1 apple or pear, 8 ounces of fresh fruit juice, 2 table-spoons raisins, 2 dates
- ▶ 1–3 servings of dairy or nondairy foods = 8 ounces low-fat milk, 4 ounces of yogurt, 8 ounces of rice or hemp milk
- ▶ 1–2 servings of animal protein = 4 ounces skinless chicken breast, 1 egg, 4 ounces wild salmon, or 3 ounces lean red meat
- ▶ 1–3 servings vegetarian protein = ½ cup beans, 4 ounces soy tempeh, 1 cup cooked lentils
- ▶ 1–2 servings of nuts, seeds, avocado, extra-virgin olive oil, flaxseed oil = 2 tablespoons daily
- ▶ Vegetables are always unlimited, with a minimum of 5 servings a day.
- ▶ Alcohol consumption is 1–3 drinks per week for women and 2–8 drinks for men.
- ▶ Recreational foods, also sometimes referred to as discretionary calories, such as chocolate, butter, honey, or other sweets should be limited to 132–512 calories per day depending on your age and body weight.

A TYPICAL DAY

Here's an example of what you might eat in a day on a whole-foods diet, based on standard portion sizes. You'll need to adjust the portions to suit your calorie needs and lifestyle.

1. **Upon rising:** Have a cup of herbal tea or fresh lemon juice in water to prepare your digestive system for the day. Keep coffee consumption to 1 cup in the morning.

2. **Breakfast:** Have ½ cup of oatmeal (not instant) or soft-cooked grains, or make a 1–2 egg omelet with cooked kale and a slice of whole-grain bread.

3. **Mid-morning snack:** 1 medium apple with ½ cup of plain yogurt and a sprinkle of cinnamon, or make a smoothie using yogurt, 1 tablespoon of green foods, ground flax meal, and hemp-seed protein powder.

4. **Lunch:** Make this the main meal of your day, with 4 ounces of animal protein, cooked broccoli or other land and sea vegetables, and fresh green salad with olive oil and apple-cider vinaigrette.

5. **Afternoon snack:** ½–1 apple with 1 tablespoon of peanut or almond butter.

6. **Dinner:** Vegetable bean or lentil soup with quinoa; grilled salmon with cooked-vegetable salad of broccoli, kale, and sweet potatoes tossed with olive oil and balsamic vinegar and topped with a tablespoon of toasted pumpkin seeds; and whole-grain bread with 1 teaspoon of nut or seed butter.

HOW VITAMINS HELP

Vitamins are essential for life—they're necessary for cell growth and to help other body systems function properly. It is essential that you get all the vitamins from your food; they work together in a synergistic way so that if one is missing your whole system is off. Oftentimes, the food you buy has traveled thousands of miles to sit on your grocery-store shelves for days or even weeks, which can deplete the food of some of its vitamins. The list of nutrients found in the twenty-five Superfoods is astounding, and when added to your daily diet these foods will help you feel energized and satisfied. For example, vitamin A is a fat-soluble vitamin that actually needs good fats and minerals to be properly absorbed. In its beta-carotene form, it neutralizes free radicals through its antioxidant properties. Numerous studies have shown that when included in the diet it can prevent bad cholesterol (LDL) from clogging the heart and coronary blood vessels. This is in addition to its ability to inhibit abnormal cell growth, strengthen the immune system, and aid in fortifying your body's cellular functions. That's a lot of things that don't happen if there's no vitamin A taken in from your food.

List of Vitamins

Familiarize yourself with the vitamins you need on a regular basis for optimal health:

- ▶ Vitamin A
- ▶ Vitamin C
- ▶ Vitamin E: alpha tocopheryl, beta, delta, and gamma
- ▶ Vitamin D (cholecalciferol)
- ▶ B Vitamins: thiamine (B1), riboflavin (B2), niacin (B3), pyridoxine (B6), folate (B9), cyanocobalamin (B12), pantothenic acid, and biotin
- ▶ Vitamin K (phylloquinone)
- ▶ Choline

*Quick tip: When you take more water-soluble vitamins than you need, small amounts are stored in body tissue—particularly the liver—but most of the excess is excreted in the urine so that they're not stored in the body in appreciable amounts.

MINERALS CAN HELP, TOO

In addition to vitamins, your body also needs the essential minerals to help in the assimilation of the vitamins. Your body utilizes over eighty minerals to help accelerate the billions of chemical reactions taking place in your body every day. There are minerals that regulate how certain vitamins are used and others that help metabolize macronutrients (e.g., proteins, carbohydrates, and fats). Some become actual components of your bones, cartilage, fingernails, and toenails, contributing to their hardness and strength (think calcium).

Nutritionally, minerals are grouped into two categories: essential minerals, also called macrominerals, and trace minerals, or microminerals. Macrominerals, such as calcium and magnesium, are needed by the body in larger amounts. Although only minute quantities of trace minerals are needed, they are nevertheless important for good health. Microminerals include boron, chromium, iron, zinc, and many others.

If you are not getting enough minerals, you may feel low on energy and experience premature aging; a diminished sense of taste, sight, and hearing; and/or symptoms of degenerative diseases such as osteoporosis, heart disease, and cancer.

DO YOU NEED FOOD SUPPLEMENTS?

Your best source for any and all essential nutrients is nutrient-dense foods. But if your diet is lacking nutrient-dense foods, you may want to take a whole-foods supplement to support your daily diet. This will help balance out any deficiencies in the processed foods you are eating as well as help with poor eating habits as you gradually improve the quality of foods you prepare.

APPLES FIGHT FREE RADICALS

I. AN APPLE A DAY KEEPS THE DOCTOR AWAY

Apples pack a whole lot of nutritional benefits as a source of antioxidants, including polyphenols, flavonoids, and vitamin C. They are a good source of fiber and potassium, which have been shown to lower your risk for heart disease and help prevent cancer.

2. KNOW THIS: POLYPHENOLS

Polyphenols are antioxidant phytochemicals that tend to prevent or neutralize the damaging effects of free radicals. Flavonoids are a class of polyphenol.

3. KEEP THE PEEL ON

Apple skin, otherwise known as apple peel, provides 2–6 times more antioxidant activity than the flesh of the apple. In particular, the skin of apples, more than most other fruits and vegetables, contains quercetin, proven to prevent unstable oxygen molecules or free radicals from damaging your cells. Free-radical damage can lead to heart disease, Type 2 diabetes, and cancer.

4. TAKE IT WITH YOU FOR A QUICK AND EASY SNACK

With only 95 calories in an average-sized apple, they are the perfect low-calorie, low-fat snack and can be used as a quick dessert, too. What's more, an apple provides 15 percent of the recommended daily dose of fiber for adults. Apples' complex carbohydrates give your body a longer, more even energy boost compared to high-sugar junk foods.

5. TRY A FUJI APPLE

Each variety of apple has its own unique skin color, and these come with a number of differences in the chemical makeup of the skin itself. This is because the phytonutrient content varies in concentration and types of polyphenols present in apple skin. The Fuji apple has the highest of total polyphenols and total flavonoid content of any apple.

But what's a phytonutrient? Also called phytochemicals, phytonutrients are components of plants thought to promote human health. Polyphenols and flavonoids are major classes of phytonutrients. These nutrients aren't essential for life in the way that other nutrients like protein, fat, vitamins, and minerals are. Apples boast polyphenols, one of the major classes of phytonutrients.

6. EAT A VARIETY OF APPLES

Because the phytonutrient makeup of the skin of each variety of apple is unique, you should eat a wide variety of apples. This ensures that you maintain a balance of all the antioxidant agents.

7. HELP YOUR HEART

According to both Finnish and Dutch researchers, catechins, a member of the flavonoid family found in apples, may reduce the risk of ischemic heart-disease mortality.

8. KEEP YOUR CHOLESTEROL IN CHECK

A diet that includes a daily dose of apples can help lower blood cholesterol thanks to pectin, the soluble fiber in apples.

9. PROTECT YOURSELF AGAINST CANCER

The flavonoids in apples may protect you against two types of cancer—bladder and lung. The flavonoids are responsible for the antimutagenicity associated with foods and beverages that protect the mucosal cells in the bladder. And based on studies done at the University of Hawaii's Cancer Research Center of Hawaii in Honolulu, the flavonoid quercetin found in apples may help protect against certain forms of lung cancer.

10. SLOW THE AGING PROCESS

Sure aging is inevitable, but by including antioxidant-rich foods such as apples into your diet you may be able to slow the process. In fact, consuming a diet high in antioxidants has a direct correlation to reduced age-related mental and physical generation, according the U.S. Department of Agriculture's Jean Mayer Human Nutrition Research Center on Aging, based at Tufts University in Boston, Massachusetts.

11. WARD OFF WRINKLES

Apples can have a positive effect on your skin and how well your skin ages. Along with a diet high in vegetables, legumes, olive oil, fruits (particularly apples), and tea, a study done by Australian researchers suggest that skin wrinkling in older people of various ethnic backgrounds due to sun overexposure may be reduced by including apples as part of a balanced whole-foods diet.

12. TRY APPLE CIDER VINEGAR

Apple cider vinegar is made from freshly pressed apple juice that is first fermented into a hard apple cider and then fermented once again into apple cider vinegar. This process allows the vinegar to retain all of the nutritional value of the apples and provides the added benefit of powerful enzymes created during the fermentation process. Health benefits associated with apple cider vinegar are as diverse as helping with weight loss to preventing ticks and fleas on your animals. You can use it to make salad dressings, homemade mayonnaise and tomato ketchup, and even as a nontoxic household cleanser, deodorizer, and disinfectant.

13. PICK THE PERFECT APPLE

When shopping for apples, pick ones that are firm, of good color, and free of soft and bruised spots.

14. STORE THEM IN THE FRIDGE

Store your apples in the crisper of the refrigerator to slow ripening and maintain crispness, as they tend to go soft ten times faster at room temperature. Also, avoid storing bruised or moldy apples with fresh ones to prevent them all from going bad.

4

15. PAIR THEM WITH PEARS

The ethylene gas produced by apples as they mature can damage leafy greens and other vegetables when stored together. On the other hand, the same ethylene can help speed the ripening of pears, bananas, peaches, and plums by placing an apple in a paper bag with the unripe fruit.

16. PASS ON THE PILLS AND EAT YOUR NUTRIENTS

Food studies out of Cornell University have consistently proven that it is the additive and synergistic effects of the phytochemicals present in fruits and vegetables that are responsible for their potent antioxidant and anticancer activities. Their findings suggest that people may gain significant health benefits by consuming more fruits and vegetables and whole-grain foods than in consuming expensive dietary supplements, which do not contain the same array of balanced complex components.

17. SUPERCHARGE YOUR SALAD

Add this apple, ginger, and carrot salad to a bed of fresh spinach or arugula leaves: Core and chop 2 apples into bite-size pieces. Place in a medium-size bowl; toss with the juice of ½ a lemon. Peel and grate 2 large carrots; add to the apples along with ¼ cup cranberries and 12 walnut halves. On the fine setting, grate a 2" piece of fresh ginger and squeeze or press to extract the juice. In a small bowl, whisk together ¼ cup extra-virgin olive oil, 1 teaspoon ginger juice, ¼ cup golden balsamic vinegar, and 1 teaspoon ume plum vinegar; pour over the apple salad. Toss to mix well and serve atop your greens.

BLUEBERRIES TO THE RESCUE

18. EAT A CUP FULL

Just 1 cup of blueberries provides you with the equivalent antioxidant content of 5 servings of carrots, broccoli, squash, and apples.

19. TRY BLUEBERRY WINE

Red wine has been touted in the media for having a beneficial effect on your heart because of the same antioxidants that blueberries contain. However, a recent study found that blueberries have 38 percent more of these antioxidants than red wine. For example, according to a study published in the *Journal of Agriculture and Food Chemistry*, 4 ounces of white wine contained .47 mmol of antioxidants; 4 ounces of red had 2.04 mmol; and the same amount of blueberry wine boasted 2.42 mmol of protective antioxidants.

20. KNOW THIS: ANTHOCYANINS

The primary force behind blueberries' superpower is the phytonutrient anthocyanin, a particular type of flavonoid—the one that gives blueberries that deep-blue pigment. It produces blue-to-red coloring in other plants (apples, grapes, blackberries, radishes, red cabbage) and flowers, too. The anthocyanin family is responsible for a long list of health benefits that are integral to how your body functions; for example, improving the integrity of support structures in the veins and entire vascular system and protecting your body against the damaging effects of free radicals and the chronic diseases associated with the aging process.

21. BOOST YOUR BONE HEALTH
The most abundant protein in your body is collagen, which is needed to form bone—cartilage, skin, and tendons, too. The anthocyanin flavonoid in blueberries is crucial for the support and stabilization of the collagen matrix.

22. HELP YOUR HEART
Several studies suggest anythocyanins help prevent heart attacks by discouraging blood clots from forming. They've also been shown to improve the integrity of support structures in the veins and entire vascular system.

23. IMPROVE YOUR VISION
The anthocyanins in blueberries also appear to improve night vision and slow macular degeneration by strengthening tiny blood vessels in the back of the eye.

24. KEEP YOUR URINARY TRACT HEALTHY
Researchers at Rutgers University in New Jersey have identified compounds in blueberries called proanthocyanins that promote urinary tract health and reduce the risk of infection by preventing bacteria from adhering to the cells that line the walls of the urinary tract. Rutgers scientist Amy Howell, PhD, explains that blueberries—like cranberries—contain these compounds that prevent the bacteria responsible for urinary tract infections from attaching to the bladder wall.

25. SHARPEN YOUR MEMORY

When it comes to brain protection, there's nothing quite like blueberries, according to neuroscientist James Joseph of Tufts University. Joseph attributes the blueberry's health benefits to its antioxidant and anti-inflammatory compounds and sees its potential for reversing short-term memory loss and forestalling many other effects of aging. In a study of reversing memory loss, the *Wall Street Journal* reported that aging rodents fed several different fruits behaved more like their younger counterparts when given blueberries to eat. The blueberries had a stronger impact on their mental functions than any of the other fruits tested.

26. BOOST YOUR FRUIT INTAKE

Based on the guidelines for getting your 5 or more servings a day of fruit and vegetables, one serving of fresh blueberries would be just ½ cup. Or, if you'd prefer juice or dried fruit, one serving of 100 percent blueberry juice is ¾ cup and one serving of dried blueberries is ¼ cup. What's more, eating only ½ cup of fresh or frozen blueberries a day will give you the antioxidant protection and antiaging properties. Top your morning cereal with a serving or two of fresh or frozen blueberries and you'll be on your way to fulfilling the dietary recommendations and better health.

27. SUPERCHARGE YOUR WAFFLES

Toss 1 cup fresh or frozen blueberries in 2 tablespoons spelt flour; set aside. Combine 2 cups spelt flour, 1½ teaspoons baking powder, ½ teaspoon salt, 1 cup of soy/rice milk, and 1 egg in a blender; purée until smooth. Pour batter into a bowl; gently stir in blueberries. Pour ¼ to ⅓ cup batter onto a heated waffle iron; cook until steam diminishes, about 1–2 minutes. Remove to a plate; top with yogurt, 1 tablespoon agave syrup, and fresh blueberries. The recipe makes 12 (4") waffles or pancakes.

28. THE ANTICANCER FRUIT

Blue and purple foods, like blueberries, can significantly lower your risk of getting certain cancers, according to the Produce for Better Health Foundation. The American Institute for Cancer Research recommends eating blueberries, too, because they are "one of the best sources of antioxidants, substances that can slow the aging process and reduce cell damage that can lead to cancer." A 2000 study in the *Journal of Food Science* looked at a particular flavonoid that inhibits an enzyme involved in promoting cancer and found that of the fruits tested, wild blueberries showed the greatest anticancer activity.

29. UP THE ANTIOXIDANT POWER OF YOUR DESSERT

Use blueberries to make a quick sauce for desserts and ice cream: heat frozen blueberries in a saucepan with a little juice or water and thicken with some cornstarch or arrowroot powder.

30. EAT BLUEBERRIES ALL YEAR

During the summer months when blueberries are abundant, buy or pick enough to freeze. To freeze blueberries, simply pour them fresh onto a baking sheet (do not wash first) and place them in the freezer. When frozen, transfer them to plastic freezer bags and store them in the freezer.

31. PREVENT BLUE BLEEDING WHEN YOU BAKE

Blueberries are wonderful in baked goods and pancakes. Fresh or frozen berries can be used, but frozen berries will discolor the batter. To prevent this blue bleeding, roll the blueberries lightly in flour before adding them to the batter. Tossing them in flour before adding them to cake batter will also keep them from sinking to the bottom of the pan.

BROCCOLI HELPS PREVENT CANCER

32. POWER UP WITH POLYPHENOLS

One of the ten most popular vegetables eaten in the United States, broccoli comes third in the amount of polyphenols it provides, with only beets and red onions containing more per serving.

33. CRUNCH ON OTHER CRUCIFERS

Broccoli is classified as *Brassica oleracea italica*, whose other members include cauliflower, kale, cabbage, collards, turnips, rutabagas, Brussels sprouts, and Chinese cabbage. The Brassica vegetables all share a common feature—a four-petal flower bearing a resemblance to the Greek cross, which explains why they are known as crucifers or cruciferous vegetables.

34. AMP UP YOUR BODY'S DETOXIFYING ENZYMES

The phytonutrient compounds in broccoli work at such a deep level that they actually signal your genes to increase production of enzymes involved in the detoxification process through which your body eliminates harmful compounds.

35. TAME TUMORS

Broccoli contains the phytonutrient sulforaphane, a compound that prevented the development of tumors by 60 percent in one study group and reduced the size of tumors that did develop in another group by 75 percent. Broccoli also contains indole-3-carbinol, a compound that helps deactivate a potent estrogen metabolite (4-hydroxyesterone) that promotes tumor growth, especially in estrogen-sensitive breast cells. Indole-3-carbinol has been shown to suppress not only breast-tumor cell growth, but also the movement of cancerous cells to other parts of the body.

36. TRY BROCCOLI SPROUTS

Broccoli sprouts have a concentrated form of the sulfur-containing phytonutrients found in broccoli, called sulforophane glucosinolate. In fact, three-day-old broccoli sprouts consistently boast 20–50 times (some research even suggests as much as 100 times) the amount of chemo-protective compounds found in mature broccoli heads, thereby offering a simple dietary means of reducing cancer risk.

37. OFFER KIDS BROCCOLI SPROUTS, EVEN WHEN THEY DON'T LIKE BROCCOLI

Children who dislike the taste of broccoli often enjoy the milder flavor of the sprouts, and they will get even more nutritional benefits. You would need to eat at least 1¼ pounds of cooked broccoli to get the same amount of protection you get from eating just 1 ounce of broccoli sprouts.

38. GROW YOUR OWN SPROUTS

In less than a week you can easily grow broccoli sprouts in your kitchen. A tablespoon of broccoli seeds will produce about 1 cup of sprouts. Start with

¼ cup of seeds to supply you with a good week's worth of sprouts. To begin, rinse the seeds and place in a sprouting or canning jar, cover with water, and let soak 8–10 hours, or overnight. With the sprouting lid in place or using a piece of cheesecloth secured to the top of the jar, drain and rinse the seeds, then drain again. Keep the jar on your counter out of direct sunlight, inverted in a large bowl and fill with cool water. Agitate the water to loosen the seed hulls. Drain the sprouts and let them dry completely. Store the sprouts in a covered container and refrigerate. They will keep for 2 weeks in the refrigerator, but for maximum benefit, eat them before that.

39. GET YOUR FOLATE
A vitamin essential for DNA synthesis and cell growth, folate is important for red blood cell formation, energy production, and the formation of amino acids. Broccoli is so rich in folate that a single cup of raw, chopped broccoli provides more than 50 milligrams of this vitamin.

40. PROTECT YOUR EYES
Broccoli provides you with the carotenoid antioxidants lutein and zeaxanthin, which, along with vitamin C, are highly beneficial for the lens and retina of the eye, to the point of protecting your eyes from free-radical damage that ultraviolet light can cause.

41. KNOW THESE: LUTEIN AND ZEAXANTHIN
These carotenoid antioxidants are related to beta-carotene. They give vegetables like carrots their orange color and add yellow pigment to plants. They are also found in large amounts in the lens and retina of the eyes, where they function as antioxidants to protect the eyes from free-radical damage.

42. REDUCE YOUR RISK OF CANCER

Eating 2 servings a day of cruciferous vegetables, including ½ cup of broccoli, may result in as much as a 50 percent reduction in the risk of certain types of cancers such as cancers of the lung, stomach, colon, and rectum, according to one study.

43. PAIR BROCCOLI WITH TOMATOES

Broccoli and tomatoes are a powerful team in preventing prostate cancer, according to a study published in *Cancer Research*. John Erdman, professor of food science and human nutrition at the University of Illinois, found that when tomatoes and broccoli are eaten together there is an additive effect due to different bioactive compounds in each food working on different anticancer pathways.

44. APPRECIATE THE SULFUR COMPOUNDS

Sure, the sulfur compounds sometimes give broccoli—and other cruciferous vegetables—a strong, and for some, unappealing odor, but the sometimes-bitter taste and smell of these vegetables is what protects them from insects and animals.

45. BEAT BLOAT AND GAS

Many people have difficulty digesting raw broccoli due to the high fiber and sulfur content of the vegetable. This can cause gas and bloating in the gastro-intestinal tract, which can lead to an embarrassing release of rather toxic-smelling fumes. Rather than eliminate these all-important cancer-fighting vegetables from your diet, make sure to cook them before eating.

46. WHEN SHOPPING FOR AND STORING BROCCOLI, HERE ARE A FEW TIPS TO REMEMBER:

► Look for the most deeply colored florets, since these contain the most phytonutrients.
► The smaller the head the better the flavor.
► Yellowing florets are signs that the broccoli is past its prime.
► Leaves on the stalks should be firm and fresh looking; wilted leaves are a sign of old broccoli.
► Broccoli will keep in the fridge crisper for up to 7 days.
► Never wash the broccoli before storing, as it can develop mold when damp.

47. GO ORGANIC!

Although it might cost a few cents more, organically grown broccoli has been shown to be higher in phytonutrients than chemically sprayed, conventionally grown varieties.

48. KEEP THE LEAVES

Do not discard the leaves, as they are also rich in nutrients. Instead, wash and cook them along with the florets.

49. SIMMER OR STEAM THE BROCCOLI

Steaming broccoli or simmering it in very little water is the best way to cook it. Keep the heat low and simmer gently, as boiled broccoli can lose more than 50 percent of its vitamin C.

QUINOA:
THE MOTHER GRAIN

50. KNOW THIS SEED

Quinoa, pronounced "keen-wah," is really a nutrient-rich seed used for thousands of years to sustain the diet of the South American Inca people. Although referred to as a grain, technically, quinoa is classified as a pseudocereal, a vegetable plant food from the Chenopodium quinoa species of the goosefoot family, the same botanical family as spinach, beets, and Swiss chard.

51. ADD PROTEIN TO YOUR DIET

Quinoa is an excellent vegetarian protein source to add to your family's diet. Considered a complete protein, quinoa provides ten essential amino acids and is packed with minerals, B vitamins, and fiber. Lifting quinoa to the status of a Superfood is extra high amounts of the amino acid lysine, which is essential for tissue growth and repair. A ¼ cup uncooked quinoa boasts nearly 6 grams of protein.

52. GO GLUTEN FREE

Good news for individuals with wheat and gluten allergies: Quinoa is an excellent replacement for processed forms of wheat such as couscous and bulgur wheat. It can easily be used in traditional Middle Eastern recipes such as couscous salad and in place of bulgur wheat in tabouli.

53. RINSE IT!

Saponins function as antinutrients and are not normally absorbed from the gut, but have been known to induce small-intestine damage or reduce intestinal absorption of some nutrients in people. Most quinoa sold commercially has already been processed to remove this coating. Nonetheless, before cooking with quinoa, place the grain in a strainer and rinse well under running water. Soaking grains for 4–8 hours in water before cooking helps make them easier to digest.

54. STAY REGULAR

As a good source of soluble and insoluble fiber, quinoa helps your bowels function properly, staving off gastrointestinal problems such as constipation, diverticulitis, colitis, and colon cancer.

55. HELP YOUR HEART

With those high doses of fiber, quinoa can now do battle with high cholesterol, heart disease, and stroke. It is when there is too much cholesterol in your blood that you can develop clogged arteries, high blood pressure, heart disease, or stroke. One study determined that for every extra 10 grams of fiber consumed a day women lowered their risk of heart disease by 19 percent.

56. MAGNIFICENT MAGNESIUM

Quinoa is also an excellent source of magnesium, an extremely important mineral essential for a number of biological processes in your body. Magnesium:

- ▶ Aids in your body's absorption of calcium
- ▶ Plays a key role in the strength and formation of bones and teeth
- ▶ Is vital for maintaining a healthy heart
- ▶ Helps stabilize the rhythm of your heart
- ▶ Helps prevent abnormal blood clotting in your heart
- ▶ Aids in maintaining healthy blood pressure levels
- ▶ Helps maintain proper muscle function by keeping them properly relaxed

57. SUBSTITUTE IT

Quinoa cooks in half the time of other grains, so swap it out when you're short on time for longer-cooking grains such as bulgur in tabouli. The ratio of water to grain is 2 cups water to 1 cup quinoa, which gives a fluffy texture good for cold salads, stir-fries, or wraps. Adding more water makes a thick, sticky mixture that can be used for making grain burgers or in wraps with other ingredients.

58. MAKE IT A SIDE SALAD

Quinoa is delicious as a cold salad mixed with chopped apple, walnuts, raisins, celery, lemon juice, and cinnamon.

59. MAKE IT A MEAL

Add some curry powder to yogurt and mix it into cooked quinoa, broccoli, and grilled chicken pieces.

60. BOOST THE FIBER IN YOUR BREAKFAST

Add cooked quinoa to your favorite pancake recipe for moist, nutritious cakes.

61. COMBINE THREE SUPERFOODS WITH THIS SALAD: QUINOA APPLE SALAD

Although you may not think to combine fruits and vegetables, in this instance the combination of tastes works perfectly together.

1. Rinse ⅓ cup quinoa in cool running water.
2. Combine 1 cup water and quinoa in a saucepan.
3. Cover, bring to a boil, and simmer on low heat until all water is absorbed.
4. Meanwhile, rinse and dry 1 bunch mesclun greens and set aside.
5. Core and chop 2 apples. Remove seeds from pepper and chop; set aside.
6. In a food processor, purée ¼ cup oil, ⅛ cup apple cider vinegar, 2 cloves garlic, 1 tablespoon agave syrup, 2 pitted dates, and ⅛ teaspoon cinnamon.
7. Add 2 tablespoons water; thin to dressing consistency.
8. Pour dressing around bottom of a large salad bowl.
9. Place mesclun in bowl. Add peppers, apples, cooled quinoa, and 1 cup chopped walnuts.
10. Toss well before serving.

DARK CHOCOLATE LOVES YOUR HEART

62. PREVENT CANCER

Chocolate may help prevent cancer. Pentameric procyanidin (pentamer), a natural compound found in cocoa, deactivates a number of proteins that likely work in concert to push a cancer cell to continually divide. Chocolate also contains polyphenol antioxidants, the same flavonoids found in green tea, a natural protection against cancer.

63. GET A DOUBLE DIP OF ANTICANCER PROTECTION

Dip strawberries in dark chocolate. Dark chocolate contains almost eight times the polyphenol antioxidants found in strawberries.

64. REMEMBER MODERATION

Keep in mind that although chocolate contains beneficial ingredients, the form it comes in can be pretty deadly to your health. Chocolate bars, cakes, cookies, and candies are often high in fat, sugar, and calories. Eat chocolate in moderation; enjoy a piece of chocolate once in a while, preferably dark chocolate with its higher flavonoid content.

65. MAKE IT A DRINK

Never fight that urge for a cup of hot chocolate again: cocoa powder ranked higher than dark chocolate, and milk chocolate came in last, according to research out of the University of Scranton that looked at the level of antioxidants in chocolate.

66. KNOW YOUR BEANS

There are three main beans in the chocolate world. The criollo bean is the superior-flavored bean reserved for only the finest, most-expensive chocolate. The more prolific forastero is the cocoa bean used for 90 percent of the world's chocolate production and for most commercial chocolate. Science went one step further and crossed the criollo with the forastero to create a high-quality hybrid cocoa bean called trinitario, know for its rich flavor.

67. FIND FAIR TRADE

Harvesting and preparing the beans is labor intensive, and various economic and governmental forces have driven the price of the bean further and further down. Some cocoa farmers have resorted to using child labor to harvest the bean and satisfy the world's sweet tooth.

68. BOOST BRAIN POWER

A compound found in cocoa—epicatechin—combined with exercise, was found to promote functional changes in a part of the brain involved in the formation of learning and memory in a study done by Salk Institute researcher Henriette van Praag and colleagues. Van Praag's work, published in the May 30, 2007, issue of the *Journal of Neuroscience*, suggests a diet rich in flavonols could help reduce the effects of neurodegenerative illnesses such as Alzheimer's disease and cognitive disorders related to aging. Epicatechin is one group of chemicals called flavonols, which have previously been shown to improve cardiovascular function and increase blood flow to the brain.

69. BOOST YOUR MOOD

Let's face it: One of the best things about chocolate is the feel-good lift you get after eating a few pieces. It can be attributed to the caffeine present in small quantities or the theobromine, a caffeine-like substance and weak stimulant present in slightly higher amounts. The combination of these two, in tandem with the other 298 chemicals present, may just provide the lift that makes your day a little better. As a matter of fact, chocolate also contains phenylethylamine, a strong stimulant related to the amphetamine family, known to increase the activity of neurotransmitters in parts of the brain that control your ability to pay attention and stay alert.

70. IMPROVE YOUR LIPID PROFILE

People who included flavonoid-rich cocoa powder and dark chocolate in their diet had a significantly higher concentration of HDL (good) cholesterol when compared with the control group, according to researchers from Penn State University who studied twenty-three people in 2001. Meanwhile, in Italy researchers found that dark chocolate may help lower blood pressure in people with hypertension. The study also found that levels of LDL (bad) cholesterol in these individuals dropped by 10 percent. They noted in *Hypertension Journal* in August 2005 that this study used a very small test group of only twenty lucky subjects, but that darker chocolate with the most concentrated cocoa proved to have the most health benefits.

71. HELP YOUR HEART

Including dark chocolate in your diet may benefit your heart, due to the phyto-chemicals mentioned earlier. The two positive effects these have on the body are the ability to block arterial damage caused by free radicals and inhibiting platelet aggregation, which could cause a heart attack or stroke. There have also been studies indicating that the flavonoids in cocoa relax the blood vessels, which inhibits an enzyme that causes inflammation.

72. IS CHOCOLATE HEALTHIER THAN TEA?

Chocolate contains up to four times the antioxidants found in tea, according to a recent study by Holland's National Institute for Public Health and Environment. The study showed that chocolate, most importantly dark chocolate, contains 53.5 mg of powerful antioxidant catechins per 100 grams. By contrast, 100 ml of black tea contains a mere 13.9 mg of catechins. To your delirious taste buds, eating chocolate may appear to be the answer to all your health problems; after all, it has so many health benefits. In order to counter the sugar, saturated fats, and artificial flavorings in commercial candy bars, many people have turned to buying chocolate in its raw, organic form and making their own sweets.

73. KNOW WHAT TO LOOK FOR WHEN BUYING CHOCOLATE

Buy only the best chocolate and beware of inexpensive chocolates blended with wax, which contain very little real cocoa butter. Inexpensive brands are made with partially hydrogenated palm oil, preservatives, and high amounts of sugar. Quality chocolate is made with real cocoa butter, the finest organic cocoa beans, minimal sugar, and an extensive refining process.

74. KEEP IT COOL TO BOOST ITS LIFESPAN

Chocolate needs to be stored at a cool temperature, in a dark place with good air circulation. Kept away from bright light, at 65°F and 50 percent humidity, unsweetened dark chocolate can last up to 10 years. In your own kitchen, dark chocolate can last up to 1 year, or 7 months for milk and white chocolate. Chocolate kept in the refrigerator should be wrapped in several layers of foil then in plastic. Allow it to return to room temperature before unwrapping; this prevents sugar bloom from occurring, which is when moisture condenses on the surface of the chocolate, drawing the sugar to the surface to crystallize and form gray or white streaks. If you store your chocolate treats in the freezer, defrost them in the refrigerator, then remove and bring to room temperature before eating.

75. SATISFY A CRAVING WITH A CHOCOLATE PEANUT BUTTER SMOOTHIE

This is the perfect recipe for when you want an instant chocolate fix. Combine 2 cups milk, 1 frozen banana, 2 heaping tablespoons of peanut butter, 1 heaping tablespoon of unsweetened chocolate powder, and your sweetener of choice in a blender; purée until smooth. Divide between 2 glasses; serve immediately.

MINERAL-RICH
SEA VEGETABLES

76. FAST FACT: WHO EATS SEA VEGETABLES

In Europe, sea vegetables have been part of life in most ocean-bordered countries such as Ireland, Scotland, Iceland, and Norway for centuries. Evidence of sea-vegetable consumption by coastal communities in New Zealand, Australia, and the Pacific Islands has also been found. Because of the high vitamin C content of sea vegetables, sea voyagers such as the Vikings and New England whalers would chew on seaweed to prevent scurvy.

77. ADD SEA VEGETABLES TO YOUR DAILY DIET

The list of nutritional benefits attributed to sea vegetables can sound too good to be true; but consider that the Japanese people, who eat the highest amounts, also have the highest longevity rates of any group of people in the world. Here's a list of what sea vegetables can add to your daily diet:

▶ Sea vegetables can contain as much as 48 percent protein.
▶ Sea vegetables are a rich source of both soluble and insoluble dietary fiber.

- The brown sea-vegetable varieties—kelp, wakame, and kombu—contain aliginic acid, which has been shown to remove heavy metals and radioactive isotopes from the digestive tract as well as strontium 90 from the bones.
- Sea vegetables contain significant amounts of vitamin A in the form of beta-carotene as well as vitamins B complex, C, and E.
- Sea vegetables are high in potassium, calcium, sodium, iron, and chloride.
- Sea vegetables provide the fifty-six minerals and trace minerals that your body requires to function properly.
- Sea vegetables contain fiber, iodine, omega-3 fatty acids, and very little fat, factors that can help with weight loss.

78. TRY ONE SEA VEGETABLE AT A TIME

Plan on buying one variety and cooking it in a few recipes before trying another. As you become more familiar with their delicious, unique flavors and their ease of preparation, begin to include a wider variety in your diet.

79. START WITH ARAME

Arame is the perfect sea vegetable to introduce to your diet, due to its mild taste and ease of preparation. It grows near the Ise peninsula of Japan in bouquets of fronds, on rocks beneath the sea. When harvested, it is chopped into thin strips, boiled, and dried.

80. USE THESE TIPS WHEN PREPARING ARAME IN YOUR KITCHEN

Before using, wash arame well to eliminate any sand or shells, and soak at least 5 minutes before cooking. Once soaked, arame can be used in stir-fry recipes, soups, and salads. Be sure to store any leftover cooked arame in the refrigerator. Once the package of dried arame has been opened, you should store it in an airtight container in a dark, cool place such as a kitchen cupboard, where it will keep indefinitely.

81. PREPARE IN MODERATION

Remember when preparing your recipe that when soaked in water, sea vegetables double in volume, while some, like wakame, expand to seven times their dried state. Read the package directions carefully or begin by soaking a small amount and increasing the amount as needed.

82. KNOW THIS SEA VEGETABLE: DULSE

The red-and-blue-colored North Atlantic sea vegetable grows as a flat, smooth frond from 6"–12" long and 6" wide, shaped like the palm of a hand. You can buy it in flake and powder forms. Dulse is high in iodine, rich in manganese, a remedy for seasickness, and a good substitute for salt.

83. MAKE DULSE A SNACK

Sauté dulse in olive oil as a topping for stemmed broccoli or as a snack by itself.

84. KNOW THIS SEA VEGETABLE: KELP

Kelp is a large, brown variety of algae, known to grow in shallow nutrient-rich ocean forests. Kelp is a Laminaria species, which are the largest sea plants in the ocean. When taken for its high iodine content, kelp is available as a supplement in powder, pill, or granular form.

85. REPLACE YOUR TABLE SALT WITH KELP

You can replace salt with kelp (dulse, too!) due to its slightly salty taste, and for the many vitamins, minerals, and especially trace minerals that it provides.

86. KNOW THIS SEA VEGETABLE: KOMBU

Kombu is a wide-leafed sea vegetable harvested wild from the northernmost island in Japan. There are several varieties of kombu, with the most popular being Japanese ma-kombu (Laminaria japonica). Look for hand-harvested kombu consisting of the most tender central part of the leaf, which has the best flavor and texture.

87. ADD SEA VEGETABLES TO BEANS

When you're cooking beans, add a little kelp or kombu. Its natural glutamic acid is a tenderizer that helps beans cook quickly and makes them more digestible.

88. KNOW THIS TERM: EXCELLENT SOURCE

When reading about foods—or looking at food labels—know that if a food is an "excellent source" of a particular nutrient, it provides 20 percent or more of the recommended daily value (RDV) for that nutrient. Foods that are a good source of a particular nutrient provide 10–20 percent of the RDV.

89. KNOW THIS SEA VEGETABLE: LAVER/NORI

Wild laver leaf is harvested from the cold North Atlantic and is the original form of nori before it is processed into thin, flat, roll-able sheets that are then used to prepare sushi rolls. Laver is actually one of the sea vegetables highest in vitamins B1, B6, B12, C, and E, and contains significant amounts of vegetable protein, fiber, iron, and other minerals and trace elements.

90. MAKE YOUR EVERYDAY MEALS MORE NUTRITIOUS

Nori is popular all over the world for its use in sushi making, but it can also be substituted for flour tortillas or pita bread. Laver plants not in sheet form are

SUPERCHARGE WITH SUPERFOODS

best lightly roasted before use, which brings out a nutty, salty flavor. And when toasted and crumbled they are especially good with noodles, rice, soups, salads, pasta, potatoes, popcorn, or hummus. Delicious crumbled onto soups, salads, pasta, potatoes, or popcorn.

91. TOAST NORI

As you already know, nori is quite versatile and toasting it and then adding it to other foods is delicious. To toast it, hold a sheet of nori by the edge and pass it over the open flame on your gas burner or electric burner set to high. Do not linger over the heat, as it will toast quickly. Do one side and then turn it over and do the other side. Now you can use it to wrap rice and vegetables or crumble it as a condiment in your soup or salad, etc.

92. KNOW THIS SEA VEGETABLE: WAKAME

Wakame is common in Atlantic waters and is black or dark green in color. It's traditionally added to miso soup, but is also good with other vegetables or in salads, stir-fry dishes, and rice dishes.

93. HEAL WITH SEA VEGETABLES

Sea vegetables have traditionally been used in Asia to treat heart disease, hypertension, cancer, and thyroid problems. The latest nutritional research shows that sea vegetables have a thermogenic effect on the metabolism, which helps the body burn its own visceral fat. Scientific researchers are working to understand how sea vegetables can be used to successfully treat disease. One recent theory proposes that consumption of laminaria (kombu) explains the low breast-cancer rate in postmenopausal Japanese women.

94. EXTEND THE LIFESPAN OF YOUR SEA VEGETABLES

Store sea vegetables in tightly sealed containers at room temperature where they can stay fresh for at least several months. When buying sea vegetables, look for those that are sold in tightly sealed packages and avoid those that have evidence of excessive moisture. Some types of sea vegetables are sold in different forms; for example, nori can be found in sheets, flakes, or powder. Choose the form that will best meet your culinary needs.

GARLIC IS NATURE'S ANTIBIOTIC

95. LEARN THIS FUN FACT

Eighteen percent of Americans consume at least one food a day containing garlic, according to data from the USDA's 1994–1996 "Continuing Survey of Food Intakes by Individuals." More garlic is eaten by Americans than French fries, ketchup, and fresh-market tomatoes.

96. ADD GARLIC TO MEATY MEALS

Because foods from the allium family help you metabolize protein efficiently they should be eaten with meals containing meat, poultry, fish, and other animal proteins. Slice the meat or fish and insert thin slices of raw garlic before cooking. Mince the raw garlic and sprinkle on top of the protein while cooking.

97. REDUCE YOUR RISK FOR HEART ATTACK AND STROKE

Eating garlic can help reduce plaque formation, which can contribute to arteriosclerosis, according to one German study published in *Toxicology Letters*. Also, clinical studies conducted by Dr. V. Petkov at the Bulgurian Academy of Sciences found that consuming garlic on a daily basis helps to lower blood pressure. All of which means that eating garlic on a regular basis also decreases your risk for heart attack and stroke.

98. CUT CANCER RISK

Eating only one clove of raw or cooked garlic daily may reduce the risk of both colon and stomach cancers, according to a study involving over 100,000 people at the University of North Carolina.

99. USE IT AS AN APHRODISIAC? DON'T EAT IT ALONE

For centuries garlic has been thought of as an aphrodisiac because eating garlic can improve blood circulation to the groin. Proper blood flow to the groin promotes a strong physical arousal for the male. To ensure intimate success, make sure that both participants are eating garlic at the same meal.

100. DON'T EAT GARLIC IN CONFINED SPACES

Eating garlic can cause intestinal flatulence in some people. A 1987 article in the *London Times* reported the plight of a French astronaut who took some snacks containing garlic on a Soviet space flight. It seems the space shuttle's air conditioning was unable to handle the astronaut's digestive special effects.

101. TRY ITS ELEPHANT COUSIN

The gigantic garlic look-alike known as elephant garlic is only a distant cousin to the garlic family. Closer to a leek in flavor, it can be roasted until soft and used as a spread on breads or whisked into a sauce calling for a hint of garlic without the overpowering taste of real garlic.

102. IMPROVE THE NUTRITIONAL BENEFITS OF GARLIC

Antiviral, antibacterial, antifungal, and antiparasitical are all properties of the simple garlic bulb. The flesh of each clove is contained within a papery skin and only releases its smell when sliced or crushed.

103. SKIP THE SUPPLEMENT

One clove of fresh garlic contains 18,300 mcg (micrograms) of allicin, while 600 mg of garlic extract only contains 3,600 mcg. This is a considerable difference and one that can determine whether a healing treatment is successful or not. Many herbalists question the efficacy of these supplements without the presence of garlic's major ingredient, but allow for it helping in certain situations. Garlic is also a good source of nutrients such as saponins, polyphenols, selenium, arginine, and vitamin C.

104. KNOW THIS TERM: ALLICIN

Allicin is a sulfur element found in garlic. It's known for its ability to cleanse and purify the body.

105. FIGHT INFECTION

The sulfur compounds in garlic are the key elements in preventing cardiovascular disease and for use as an antibiotic. In one study, garlic was tested on mice against an antibiotic-resistant strain of staphylococci. The results showed the garlic had protected the mice against the pathogen and significantly reduced any inflammation.

106. HELP YOUR HEART

The heart-related ailments that garlic is claimed to help includes:

► Atherosclerosis: helps to open the blood vessels in the body

► Cardiovascular disease: sulfur compounds reduce the formation of blood clots

► High cholesterol: helps reduce levels of low-density lipoprotein (LDL or bad) cholesterol

► High blood pressure: using powdered garlic helps lower blood pressure

107. WARD OFF MOSQUITOES

Garlic is thought to possibly act as an insect repellent.

108. FIND FRESH GARLIC

Many manufacturers store garlic for up to 6 months after it has been harvested and up to a year under controlled storage, so buying fresh from a local garlic grower is ideal, if possible.

109. COMBINE THREE SUPERFOODS INTO ONE DELICIOUS SUM-MER RECIPE: CUCUMBER GAZPACHO

Chop the vegetables in the food processor according to your preference for texture. Some may want a smoother soup while others will want it with bigger chunks. This is where you can make this dish to suit your individual tastes and desires.

1. Peel, trim, quarter lengthwise, seed, and chop 5 medium cucumbers. Hold back a cup of chopped cucumber for garnish.

2. In a food processor, process remaining cucumber in batches, scraping sides. Remove cucumbers to a bowl and set next to food processor.

3. Core, seed, and chop 1 medium sweet onion, 2 large red peppers, and 1 medium jalapeño; pulse chop in food processor. Add to cucumbers.

4. In processor, purée 4 medium cloves of garlic, ¾ cup fresh mint leaves, ½ cup parsley, 2 cups plain organic yogurt, 1 teaspoon sea salt, and 3 tablespoons white-wine vinegar. While machine is running, add ¾ cup extra-virgin olive oil slowly through feed slot.

5. Fold into cucumber mixture; add 1 cup vegetable stock and 1 cup water, stirring to combine.

6. Adjust seasonings. Refrigerate until chilled. Serve topped with ½ cup toasted pine nuts, chopped cucumber, and minced parsley.

AVOCADOS
ARE FULL OF GOOD FAT

110. BOOST YOUR FAT INTAKE?

Surprisingly, it's the fat in avocados (the monounsaturated form called oleic acid) that has been show to help lower cholesterol, prevent heart disease and arteriosclerosis, and lower your risk for cancer.

111. MOISTURIZE DRY SKIN

Fifty percent of the fat in avocados is oleic acid. This beneficial fat and all of the nutrients it contains keeps your body well oiled and can be used internally or externally as a skin conditioner and moisturizer.

112. DECORATE YOUR MEAL

Use chopped avocados as a garnish for black beans and rice, vegetarian bean tacos, or in burritos or wraps.

113. MAKE YOUR AVOCADO INTO A DRESSING

You can add avocado to a tofu-based dressing recipe for extra richness and added color.

114. PREPARE AN AVOCADO IN THREE EASY STEPS

Opening an avocado and removing the seed is the first step in using this super-delicious fruit.

1. Begin by cutting around a ripe avocado lengthwise and twisting the two halves to separate.
2. To remove the seed, take a knife and whack it sharply against the seed then twist slightly. The seed will separate from the flesh and you will be able to easily remove it. Be careful taking the seed off the knife, as it can be a bit slippery.
3. At this point, you can either peel the skin from the flesh and cut the flesh into long slices or cubes or, holding the avocado half in one hand, score the flesh with a knife and use a spoon to gently scoop the flesh onto a plate or bowl. To make rings or crescents, cut around the avocado cross-wise before peeling then peel the slices. Cut the rings in half to make crescent shapes. To make avocado balls, you can scoop the avocado meat from the unpeeled half-shell with a melon-ball cutter or round spoon.

115. KNOW THE DIFFERENCE BETWEEN A SUMMER AND WINTER AVOCADO

There are many varieties of avocado, and being a year-round fruit they can vary in size and shape from season to season. The winter avocado is thin skinned and pear shaped with a deep forest-green color and weighs 6–16 ounces. The summer season produces more varieties, with skins that can be thick or thin, rough or smooth, with many pear shaped and some round and plump. The skin color can vary from green to almost black, with a weight variation of 10–40 ounces.

40

116. GROW YOUR OWN

You can easily grow an avocado tree by placing four strong, sharp-tipped tooth-picks about 1" above the wide base of the seed. Place the wide end of the seed into a glass of water, balancing the toothpicks along the rim of the glass. Keep the water level constant until the seed sprouts roots and shoots, then plant it in soil.

117. KNOW THIS TERM: HASS AVOCADO

There are two varieties of avocados available in the United States, and each differs in size, appearance, quality, and susceptibility to cold weather. The Hass variety is grown in California and has a tough, bumpy skin and buttery consistency. It is presently the most popular type. It was named for Rudolph Hass, a Wisconsin mailman who retired to Pasadena and obtained a patent for the Hass avocado tree in 1935. They are rich in healthy monounsaturated oil, with 18–30 percent oil in each avocado.

118. CUT BACK ON FAT WITH THE WEST INDIAN AVOCADO

The West Indian avocado is from Florida. It's light green and larger and juicier than the Hass variety, but it is less buttery and considerably lower in oil. The Florida avocado contains just 3–5 percent oil and roughly 25–50 percent less fat than the Hass variety.

119. ENJOY AVOCADO IN MODERATION

It's tempting to eat a whole, ripe avocado at a single sitting, but be aware that one whole California avocado has over 300 calories and 35 grams of fat, 8.5 grams being monounsaturated fat. On a healthier note, it also boats high amounts of vitamin E, fiber, folate, potassium, and magnesium.

120. HELP YOUR HEART
The all-important mineral magnesium—as well as potassium—helps regulate blood pressure and prevent circulatory diseases including high blood pressure, stroke, and heart disease. Just 1 cup of avocado contains 23 percent of the daily value for folate, which when combined with the monounsaturated fats and potassium decreases your chances of cardiovascular disease and stroke.

121. MORE MIGHTY MAGNESIUM BENEFITS
Ounce for ounce, avocados provide more magnesium than the twenty most commonly eaten fruits. Magnesium is an essential nutrient for healthy bone and cardiovascular systems (particularly in the regulation of blood pressure and cardiac rhythms), prevention of migraines, and prevention of Type 2 diabetes.

122. CUT YOUR CHOLESTEROL
Avocados are rich in beta-sitosterol, a so-called phytosterol, which is the plant equivalent of cholesterol in animals. The avocado is one of the best sources of beta-sitosterol you can obtain from whole foods. Because beta-sitosterol is so similar to cholesterol, it competes for absorption with cholesterol and wins, thus lowering the amounts of cholesterol in your bloodstream. One study found that after seven days on a diet that included avocados there were significant decreases in both total and LDL (bad) cholesterol, as well as an 11 percent increase in HDL (good) cholesterol. What's more, based on both animal and laboratory studies, beta-sitosterol also appears to inhibit excessive cell division, which may play a role in preventing cancer-cell growth.

123. BOOST YOUR NUTRIENT UPTAKE

Perhaps the most interesting research on avocados demonstrates that it is a powerful nutrient booster and can actually improve your body's ability to absorb nutrients. This was demonstrated in two separate studies. In one study, adding about ½ an avocado to a mixed green and grated-carrot salad increased the absorption of alpha carotene by 8.3 times, beta-carotene by 13.6 times, and lutein by 4.3 times in the subjects who ate the salad compared with the absorption rate of the same salad without avocado. In a second study, adding a medium avocado to a serving of salsa increased the absorption of lycopene 4.4 times and the absorption of beta-carotene 2.6 times compared with eating the salsa without the avocado. Both studies showed that the healthy monounsaturated fat in the avocado caused a significant increase in the absorption of the fat-soluble carotenoid phytonutrients in the meal.

124. FIGHT PROSTATE CANCER

Recent research indicates that the avocado is a potent warrior in the fight against prostate cancer. They contain the highest amount of carotenoid lutein of any commonly eaten fruit as well as carotenoids including zeaxanthin, alpha-carotene, and beta-carotene and significant amounts of vitamin E, all beneficial for maintaining a healthy prostate. One study showed that an extract of avocado containing these carotenoids and tocopherols inhibited the growth of prostate cancer cells. Interestingly, when researchers used lutein (the carotenoid in tomatoes) alone, the cancer cells were unaffected, thus demonstrating once again that it's the synergy of health-promoting nutrients in whole foods that makes the difference.

125. PICK A TREE-RIPENED AVOCADO

A ripe avocado is slightly soft, but should have no dark sunken spots or cracks. A good test for ripeness is to stick a toothpick into the stem end; the fruit is ready to eat if the pick glides in easily. An avocado with a slight neck, rather than rounded on top, was probably tree ripened and will have better flavor.

126. TRY THIS: RIPEN AN AVOCADO

If you were only able to find an unripe avocado, you can ripen it in a paper bag or fruit basket at room temperature within a few days. Avocados should not be refrigerated until they are ripe. Once ripe, they can be kept refrigerated for up to a week.

127. STORE IT WITH THE SEED

Any leftover avocado can be placed in a container with the avocado seed and stored in the refrigerator. The seed will help slow down the browning of the flesh. You can also sprinkle the exposed surface of the avocado with lemon juice to prevent the browning that can occur when the flesh comes in contact with oxygen in the air.

128. SPICE UP YOUR GUACAMOLE

The unique flavor of cumin complements the avocado without being overbearing. This dip is perfect with a south-of-the-border menu or spread on warm tortilla chips. Peel and seed 2 medium, ripe avocados; in a medium-size bowl mash the meat until smooth. Add 2 tablespoons lemon juice, 2 tablespoons extra-virgin olive oil, ⅛ teaspoon garlic powder, 1 tablespoon chives, 1 teaspoon sea salt, and 1 teaspoon ground cumin; mix to combine thoroughly. Cover and keep in the refrigerator until ready to serve. Letting this dip sit for 15 minutes helps blend the flavors.

PARSLEY:
THE BLOOD CLEANSER

129. TAKE THE TIME TO CHOP AND INCLUDE PARSLEY IN YOUR DIET

Why? Here are the beneficial properties of parsley:

▶ **Diuretic:** helps reduce water retention and swelling in your limbs and enlarged glands
▶ **Carminative:** improves circulation and stimulation to body parts
▶ **Expectorant:** helps excrete excess mucus from the lungs
▶ **Nervine:** used to feed and tone the nerves
▶ **Tonic:** used to strengthen blood and organs

130. FIND FRESH PARSLEY

It takes 12 pounds of fresh parsley to make 1 pound of dried. If you have a choice, use fresh parsley, which provides more flavor and health benefits than dried and requires little more than a quick mincing with a knife or snip of the scissors.

131. TRY THIS: FLAT-LEAF PARSLEY

Known as Italian parsley, it has a distinctive flat, saw-toothed leaf and a stronger, sweeter flavor than the curly variety. The flat-leaf variety is far more delicate and lacy and gets very leggy. It grows to about 18" in height and seeds in its second year.

132. GO MILDER

Curly leaf (Petroselinum crispum) is milder tasting than the flat leaf. This variety lends itself to working as a team with other herbs. Its compact, dense, bright-green leaves tend to make it an attractive edging or container plant. Curly leaf can be used in just about any dish, bringing both color and just the right amount of flavor to the recipe. This variety grows as high as 12" tall and needs full sun and rich composted soil to grow.

133. SPICE UP YOUR PESTO

To make healthy, great-tasting pesto, add a generous amount of parsley to the traditional basil, olive oil, garlic, pine nuts, and Parmesan cheese recipe. The flat-leaf variety of parsley can be a bit strong and tends to overpower the flavor of the basil, so use the curly leaf instead. Bonus: The parsley helps neutralize your breath from the effects of eating raw garlic.

134. GO OLD SCHOOL

Pesto was born in the northern Italian city of Genoa. Pesto is the Genoese adjective meaning "pounded" or "crushed," from the Latin root for pestle, as in mortar and pestle. Today, it can be made quickly in an electric food processor, but if you ever have the time, try working the ingredients by hand and see if you notice a difference in taste and quality.

135. TRY THIS RECIPE: WALNUT PARSLEY PESTO

1. Add ⅓ cup fresh walnuts to the grinding bowl or processor; grind to a pulp.
2. Add 3 cloves garlic to grinding bowl or processor; continue to grind.
3. Add 2 cups curly leaf parsley (no stems) and 2 cups fresh basil leaf in batches, along with 1 tablespoon of extra-virgin olive oil; continue to grind.
4. As ingredients break down, continue to add olive oil by tablespoons up to ½ cup and ½ teaspoon sea salt until you have a thick paste.
5. Adjust consistency by adding more oil to make a sauce that is not too thick yet not loose and runny.

136. BE PATIENT

Starting a parsley plant from seed requires a long gestation period. Begin by soaking the seeds overnight, then place in potting soil and keep in a warm place. It could take several weeks, so patience is called for here. Once they sprout, you can put them on a warm, sunny windowsill, water them regularly, and let them grow. You can replant once they are strong enough for the outdoors or pot them and keep them indoors or on the porch.

137. GET MORE VITAMIN C

Did you know that parsley has a higher vitamin C content than citrus? And because vitamin C can be used to treat internal inflammation, parsley is an excellent ingredient in remedies to treat this problem. It can also protect against free-radical damage. Free radicals contribute to the development and progression of a wide variety of diseases including atherosclerosis, colon cancer, diabetes, and asthma. Individuals who consume a diet high in vitamin C foods have less of a risk for these kinds of disease. Parsley is a nutrient-dense herb, boasting more than just C: it contains vitamins A and K, iodine, iron, and chlorophyll.

138. KEEP IT IN SIGHT

If you will be using your parsley over just a few days, clip the tips of the stems and arrange in a glass of water. Set it on your counter where you can reach over and snip enough to garnish your food. Oftentimes, out of sight out of mind can hold true for using fresh herbs in your cooking. If the parsley is there in front of you, you are more likely to find a way to use it. When keeping your fresh parsley for a week or longer it should be covered and stored in the refrigerator.

139. PRESERVE YOUR PARSLEY

To freeze fresh parsley, wash off any sand or dirt and shake to dry. Place in freezer bags and into your freezer. Try to use frozen parsley within 2 months. To dry your own parsley, bundle fresh-cut stems and wrap the ends with twine. Hang the bunch of parsley upside down from a rafter or window frame. When completely dry and crisp, gently remove the parsley leaves, place in a glass jar, and seal tightly. Store in a cool, dry place out of the sunlight.

140. UNITE SUPERFOODS: HERBED AND ROASTED VEGETABLES

Serve Walnut Parsley Pesto with your favorite pasta or on top of these roasted vegetables.

1. Preheat oven to 400°F.
2. Chop 1 onion, 1 large zucchini, 2 cups broccoli florets, 2 cups cauliflower florets, and 7 small red-skin potatoes into medium-size pieces. Trim 1 pound green beans but leave long.

48

3. Place vegetables in a large bowl; toss with ¼ cup olive oil to lightly coat.

4. Spread vegetables out on a baking sheet; roast uncovered 20 minutes, or until potatoes are tender.

5. When vegetables are done move them to a platter and top each serving with a dollop of Walnut Parsley Pesto.

WILD SALMON
KEEPS YOUR SKIN YOUNG

141. EAT LIKE AN ESKIMO

After observing that the Eskimo population had a diet rich in fish oil and a low rate of heart disease, scientists began to take a serious interest in omega-3 fatty acids. Salmon is only one source for the two types of omega-3s: DHA (docosahexaenoic acid) and EPA (eicosapentaenoic acid). It is the omega-3 fatty acids in salmon that put this fish at the top of the Superfoods chart, but that's not all; it is also high in vitamin D, selenium, protein, and B vitamins.

142. PUT A LITTLE VARIETY INTO YOUR DIET

Other sources of omega-3 fatty acids include fatty fish like mackerel, lake trout, herring, sardines, and albacore tuna. The American Heart Association (AHA) recommends eating fish (particularly fatty fish) at least two times a week.

143. BOOST YOUR BABY'S BRAIN POWER

Omega-3 fatty acids are required for normal brain development of fetuses during pregnancy and for the first two years of life. If mother and infant are deficient in omega-3 fatty acids, the infant's immune and nervous systems may not develop correctly.

144. FIGHT INFLAMMATION
Omega-3s are potent anti-inflammatory agents that help curb an overactive immune system, and thus are helpful in the treatment of autoimmune diseases such as rheumatoid arthritis, chronic inflammatory bowel disease, Crohn's disease, and psoriasis. They also prolong the survival of those who suffer from them.

145. KNOW THIS: HOW SALMON GET THEIR 3S
Wild salmon thrive on zooplankton (tiny, single-celled organisms), which are a rich source of omega-3 fatty acids.

146. GO WILD!
Today, most salmon in the food markets are farmed and there is a wide variation in price between inexpensive farmed salmon and expensive fresh Alaskan salmon. The year-round demand for salmon far exceeds its availability. In order to fulfill this demand, farms for raising salmon in captivity were created. Farm-raised salmon contains less of the heart-healthy omega-3 fatty acids because they're not always fed the marine diet that produces high amounts of omega-3 fatty acids. What's more, they may have higher levels of chemical contaminants and are most likely genetically engineered for size and color enhanced to make the flesh more appealing to a discerning public.

In a study appearing in *Environmental Health Perspectives* in May 2005, the research team reported that the levels of chlorinated pesticides, dioxins, PCBs, and other contaminants are up to ten times greater in farm-raised salmon than in wild Pacific salmon and that salmon farmed in Europe are more contaminated than salmon from South and North American farms.

147. KNOW WHEN FARM-RAISED IS AN OKAY CHOICE

For a middle-aged man who has had a heart attack and doesn't want to have another one, the risks from pollutants are minor and the omega-3 benefits him in a way that far outstrips the relatively minor risks from the pollutants, according to Steven Schwager, Cornell associate professor. However, for the younger generation, who are at risk of a lifetime accumulation of pollutants, and pregnant women, who are at risk for birth defects and IQ diminution and other kinds of damage to the fetus, those risks are great enough that they outweigh the benefits.

148. KNOW WHERE TO BUY FARMED SALMON

Research suggests there are regional differences in contaminants in farmed salmon, with Chilean salmon showing the lowest levels and European (particularly Scottish) farmed salmon showing the highest levels. They maintain that careful consumers with a history of heart disease should choose farmed salmon from Chile for their high omega-3 content and relatively lower level of contaminants and that farmed salmon from North America would be a better second choice than European farmed salmon.

149. KNOW WHERE NOT TO BUY FARMED SALMON

Researchers suggests that consumers should not eat farmed fish from Scotland, Norway, and eastern Canada more than three times a year; from Maine, western Canada, and Washington state more than three to six times a year; and from Chile more than about six times a year.

150. HOW MUCH SALMON IS SAFE?

Wild chum salmon can be consumed safely as often as once a week; pink salmon, sockeye, and coho about twice a month; and Chinook just once a month.

151. BE HAPPY

Because over 60 percent of your brain is fat, your mental health is affected by your intake of the essential fatty acids. Omega-3 fatty acids not only promote your brain's ability to regulate mood-related signals, they are crucial constituents of brain-cell membranes and are needed for normal nervous system function, mood regulation, and attention and memory functions. Cultures that have high omega-3 consumption from eating fish have far less mental depression than Americans whose diets are dominated by omega-6 fatty acids. In fact, in one epidemiological study, fish consumption was the most significant variable in comparing levels of depression and coronary heart disease.

152. HELP YOUR HEART

How omega-3 fatty acids reduce cardiovascular disease (CVD) risk is still being studied. Epidemiologic and clinical trials have shown that omega-3 fatty acids reduce CVD incidence. The ideal amount to take isn't clear, but evidence from prospective secondary prevention studies suggests that taking EPA+DHA ranging from 0.5–1.8 grams per day (either as fatty fish or supplements) significantly reduces deaths from heart disease and all other causes. For alpha-linolenic acid, a total intake of 1.5–3 grams per day seems beneficial. And randomized clinical trials have shown that omega-3 fatty-acid supplements can reduce cardiovascular events (death, nonfatal heart attacks, nonfatal strokes). However, more studies are needed to confirm and further define the health benefits of omega-3 fatty-acid supplements for preventing a first or subsequent cardiovascular event. However, other research has shown that omega-3s decrease risk of arrhythmias, which can lead to sudden cardiac death; decrease triglyceride levels; decrease growth rate of atherosclerotic plaque; and lower blood pressure (slightly).

153. EAT SALMON FOR YOUR EYES

In the Nurses' Health Study, conducted by Harvard University, those who ate fish four or more times a week had a lower risk of age-related macular degeneration than those who ate three or fewer fish meals per month.

154. TRY CANNED SALMON

Use canned salmon to make salmon burgers: mash with egg and breadcrumbs, then grill. Or make it the way you do canned tuna, with mayonnaise, onion, and celery. Replace the beef in meatloaf with it. Lastly, combine salmon with corn kernels, eggs, onion, and bread crumbs to make croquettes.

155. COOK FRESH SALMON EASILY

Because salmon is versatile and adaptable to any cooking method, you can bake, broil, poach, grill, boil, sauté, fry, or steam it. Salmon can be cooked with a honey-citrus glaze; with brown sugar and pecans; topped with minced garlic and olive oil; sprinkled with herbs de Provence and butter; poached in lemon juice or white wine; grilled with parsley butter; slathered with pesto; or baked with dill.

BEANS LOWER CHOLESTEROL

156. EAT THE RECOMMENDED AMOUNT

One of the major recommendations of the 2005 Dietary Guidelines for Americans was for people to include 3 cups of beans on a weekly basis. The guidelines classify beans as a vegetable and as a nonmeat protein source because they contain nutrients found in both of the respective food groups.

157. START OFF SLOW!

Allow your digestive system to get used to beans by beginning with lentils and gradually adding beans to your diet. Then begin with beans that are easier to digest such as navy, great northern, aduki, or black beans.

158. EASE YOUR DIGESTION

Because they are a protein-starch combination, beans can cause digestive gas, which can be neutralized by using ginger, kombu (sea vegetable), or bay leaf in the cooking process. Look for Eden brand organic beans in your natural-foods store. They cook the beans with the seaweed kombu, which helps reduce the gaseous qualities in the beans while replacing some of the mineral content destroyed in the heating process.

159. BITE INTO HISTORY

Beans are one of the oldest recorded foods in history. Archeological digs have unearthed beans and lentils 5,000 years old in the Eastern Mediterranean, Mesopotamia, the Egyptian pyramids, Hungarian caves, the British Isles, the American continents, and up into India and the Middle East.

160. KITCHEN TOOL TO TRY: PRESSURE COOKER

The average cooking time for beans is 1½–2 hours when simmered on the stovetop. Using a pressure cooker can reduce the cooking time by half. For optimal digestion, be sure to presoak the beans 6–8 hours before cooking.

161. BRANCH OUT

There are many more than the commonly used kidney, garbanzo, or lentil beans awaiting your discovery:

Anasazi (a-na-SAH-zee) beans: indigenous to the Native American Navajo tribes, anasazi means "ancient one." Cultivated since AD 1100, this heirloom bean has a sweet flavor, is fast cooking, and is reputed to cause less flatulence than other bean varieties. They can be used in place of pinto beans to make delicious refried beans.

Azuki beans: also called aduki or black aduki beans. Usually a small red bean, with the less-common cousin being the black azuki. These beans have a sweet-sour flavor, are easy to digest, and cook faster than other beans. For healing purposes, they detoxify the body, reduce swelling, and cleanse stagnant blood conditions.

Black turtle beans: a member of the kidney-bean family, they are most often found in Latin American cuisine cooked with bay leaf, basil, onion, and green pepper. Helps support the kidneys and reproductive organs, acts as a diuretic (dispels fluids), and lessens the effects of urinary problems and menopausal hot flashes.

Cannellini, navy, and great northern beans: smooth-textured, kidney-shaped white beans with a sweet, nutty flavor; they are mostly used in soups and salad recipes. They are thought to be beneficial to the lungs and help the elasticity and vibrancy of the skin.

Mung beans: commonly used to make the Indian dish dahl, mung beans are a highly nutritious bean and easy to prepare. They are beneficial to the liver and gall bladder and act as a diuretic, helping to reduce swelling in the body. With 14 grams of protein, 55 grams of calcium, and 97 grams of magnesium in 1 cup of cooked mung beans, you cannot afford to live without this Superfood. Check the end of this book for a delicious mung-bean stew your family will love.

Lentils: a good source of fiber, B vitamins, and protein without any fat. With 1 cup of cooked lentils you get 230 calories, 18 grams of protein, and 16 grams of fiber, all beneficial for your heart, circulation, adrenals, and kidneys.

162. REDUCE YOUR RISK FOR HEART DISEASE

Eating high-fiber foods such as beans and lentils helps prevent cardiovascular disease, according to a study published in the *Archives of Internal Medicine*. In this study, almost 10,000 American adults were followed for nineteen years. Those eating the most fiber—21 grams per day—had a 12 percent reduced risk for developing coronary heart disease (CHD) and 11 percent reduced risk for developing cardiovascular disease (CVD) compared to those eating the least fiber—5 grams—daily. Those eating the most water-soluble dietary fiber fared even better, with a 15 percent reduction in risk of CHD and a 10 percent risk reduction in CVD.

163. FILL UP ON FIBER

Beans and lentils are the perfect food for individuals with hypoglycemia and diabetes to have on a daily basis. The fiber content helps stabilize blood-sugar levels while providing a steady, slow-burning source of energy.

164. BE BUDGET FRIENDLY

For the lowest cost, buy dried beans in bulk and cook in large batches, freezing some to be used later. When buying in bulk, move the beans from plastic bags to glass mason jars and store in a cool, dry place. Try to use them as soon as possible because as dried beans get old, they toughen up and will not cook completely.

165. KEEP SALT IN CHECK

If you are reluctant to cook your beans, you can buy canned organic beans and use those, but just make sure to look for low-salt brands and rinse them well before using.

166. COOK BEANS IN FIVE EASY STEPS

The basic principle for cooking all beans is the same, no matter how you plan to use them in a recipe.

1. Before cooking, pick through the beans and remove any stones, broken beans, or other bits of debris.
2. Place the beans and enough water to cover in a large, heavy pot. Cover and allow to soak overnight or during the day. Drain the water and add fresh water before cooking.
3. To help reduce the flatulence properties, add a small piece of kombu seaweed or ginger to the water. Bring water to a hard boil, reduce the heat, and let the beans simmer until tender, usually about 45–50 minutes. Skim any foam that rises to the surface. At this point, you can add vegetables and seasonings such as potatoes, carrots, peppers, basil, and bay leaf.
4. About 15 minutes before the beans are done add the salt and any acidic ingredients like tomatoes. The salt helps bring out the full flavor of the beans, but adding salt and acidic foods too early inhibits the water's ability to penetrate the beans, leaving them hard and tough no matter how long you boil them.
5. When the beans are soft and tender, adjust the seasonings as needed.

167. MAKE THIS NUTRIENT-RICH GRAIN SALAD

For grain salads, the longer it marinates the better the flavors are absorbed by the ingredients. Make it the night before and take some to work for lunch the next day. Bring this salad along for a potluck meal and watch how your friends enjoy something new and delicious.

1. In a medium saucepan, combine 1 cup quinoa, 2 cups water, and ½ teaspoon sea salt. Cover, bring to a boil, reduce heat to low, and simmer until all water is absorbed, about 20 minutes.
2. When done, spoon into a large bowl and allow to cool.
3. Meanwhile, grate 1 carrot, slice 2 green onions, toast ⅓ cup pumpkin seeds, mince ½ cup parsley leaves, and rinse 1 (14-ounce) can of beans.
4. When quinoa is cool, add carrots, green onions, pumpkin seeds, black beans, and parsley; mix well.
5. In a small bowl, whisk together the juice of 1 lemon, 1 clove minced garlic, 2 tablespoons apple cider vinegar, 3 tablespoons extra-virgin olive oil, and salt.
6. Add vinaigrette; mix completely and allow to marinate a few minutes before serving.

168. FILL UP ON FIBER WITH THESE TWO-BEAN CHILI WRAPS

Here is a vegetarian chili that tastes great and introduces you to the soy food called tempeh. Made from fermented soybeans, tempeh is high in B vitamins and is an excellent protein substitute for saturated fatty meats.

1. In a large saucepan, heat 2 tablespoons olive oil; sauté 6 cloves garlic and 1 chopped onion until soft.
2. Add 2 teaspoons cumin, 1 teaspoon turmeric, and 1 teaspoon cayenne; cook until roasted, 1 minute.
3. Add 16-ounces tempeh; cook 3 minutes.
4. Add 1 chopped zucchini, 1 chopped red pepper, and 1 can (14-ounce) diced tomatoes; stir well.

5. Add 1 can (15-ounce) kidney beans, 1 can (15-ounce) cannellini beans, both drained and rinsed, and ½ cup kalamata olives; stir well.

6. Add a pinch of stevia and sea salt to taste.

7. Cover, reduce heat, and simmer 20 minutes.

8. Lightly heat 6 whole-grain tortillas and spoon a portion of 2 cups cooked brown rice along center of each. Top with chili, part of 1 avocado, and grated Romano or goat cheese.

9. Sprinkle with chopped parsley, roll, and serve.

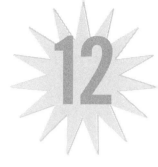

KALE: A POWERHOUSE OF NUTRIENTS

169. LEARN THIS FUN FACT
Pizza Hut is thought to be the largest consumer of kale in the United States, specifically using it to garnish their salad bars.

170. DETOXIFY NATURALLY
Kale—and other Brassica vegetables—contain a potent glucosinolate phytonutrient, which actually boosts your body's detoxification enzymes, clearing potentially carcinogenic substances more quickly from your body.

171. FEND OFF COLON CANCER
Researchers at Rutgers University found that animals fed sulforaphane developed smaller tumors that grew more slowly and had less risk of developing intestinal polyps the more sulforaphane they were given. What's more, a Netherlands Cohort Study on Diet and Cancer showed that over the course of six years, 100,000 people benefitted with a 25 percent lower risk of colorectal cancers from eating vegetables, while those eating the most cruciferous vegetables, such as kale, did almost twice as well, dropping their cancer risk by 49 percent.

172. TRY A VARIETY OF CANCER-FIGHTING VEGGIES

More common members of the prestigious Brassica family of vegetables include: cabbage, broccoli, Brussels sprouts, cauliflower, kale, collards, mustard leaves, rapini, bok choy, and broccoli rabe. With so many choices, take advantage of having a different variety each day of the week.

173. GO JURASSIC!

Today, the two most common varieties are the dinosaur kale and the ornamental kale, also known as salad savoy. The dinosaur kale was first discovered in Italy at the end of the nineteenth century, while the ornamental kale was first cultivated in California in the 1980s.

174. STRENGTHEN YOUR BONES

With all the buzz about getting enough calcium, many people are taking supplements with the promise that they can avoid losing bone density. What you should know is that eating calcium-rich foods is a much better way to strengthen your bones than getting your calcium in pill form. According to a study from Washington University in St. Louis, women who consumed an average of 830 mg (milligrams) of calcium per day in the foods they ate tested higher for bone mineral densities (BMDs) than women who took 1,033 mg of calcium in supplement form. If you feel, however, that you are unable to eat the required amounts of calcium-rich foods, the study also showed that women who received at least 70 percent of their calcium from food plus took a calcium supplement tested highest in BMDs, with an intake of 1,620 mg of calcium per day.

175. ABSORB MORE CALCIUM WITH KALE

Although you may think that dairy products are the best and only sources for ingesting calcium, there is a wide range of foods that actually allow you to digest and absorb your calcium better than pasteurized dairy products, including kale. Just by including kale and other calcium-rich vegetables in your weekly diet, you will be receiving the calcium your body requires for strong bones, proper estrogen metabolism, blood clotting, nerve conduction, muscle contraction, enzyme activity, and cell membrane function.

176. PREVENT PROSTATE CANCER

In a study conducted at the Fred Hutchinson Cancer Research Center in Seattle of over 1,200 men, those eating 28 servings of vegetables a week lowered their risk of developing prostate cancer by 35 percent, while those including just 3 or more servings of cruciferous vegetables a week lowered their risk by a whopping 44 percent.

177. LOWER LUNG CANCER RISK

Kale is thought to ease lung congestion. A study of Chinese women in Singapore, a city in which high air-pollution levels put stress on the detoxification capacity of residents' lungs, found that in nonsmokers, eating cruciferous vegetables lowered risk of lung cancer by 30 percent. In smokers, regular cruciferous vegetable consumption reduced lung cancer risk an amazing 69 percent!

178. SHIELD YOUR EYES NATURALLY

Rather than looking to supplements for your protection, research suggests that food sources are your best bet for eye-protective antioxidants. Lutein and zeaxanthin are found in the eye's macula in a ratio similar to that found in foods. Lutein is most effective when accompanied by other antioxidants, such as fruits and vegetables. The Eye Disease Case-Control Study through the National Eye Institute found that those with the highest blood levels of lutein and zeaxanthin, two antioxidants found in kale, were 70 percent less likely to develop age-related macular degeneration (ARMD) than those with the lowest levels. Individuals who consumed leafy green vegetables such as kale, spinach, and collard greens for 5 or more servings per week had a 43 percent less risk of ARMD than those who consumed the greens once a month or less. What's more, kale also guards your eyes against forming cataracts. In the Nurse's Health Study, the nurses who ate cooked greens more than twice a week had one-third fewer cataracts requiring surgery than those who ate them less than once a month.

179. GO ORGANIC

To get the most benefit from your kale, be sure to choose organically grown varieties, as their phytonutrient levels are higher than conventionally grown kale.

180. KEEP IT NUTRITIOUS

Preparing your greens using one of these two methods—water-sauté or steam—has been shown to retain the most phytonutrients and maximize their availability to your body. Try to use it up within 3 days to retain the nutrients and freshness.

> **Water-sauté method**: Wash and drain the kale then run a sharp knife along the stem to remove the leaves. Pour ½" of water into a large skillet and add the kale leaves. Cover, bring to a simmer, and cook until tender,

68

about 6–7 minutes. Remove kale to a colander and rinse with cool water to stop the cooking process. Gently squeeze out any water and chop the kale.

Steam method: Place ½" of water in a large saucepan and arrange a steamer basket on the inside of the pan. Add the kale, cover, and bring to a boil. Reduce heat and allow to steam until kale is tender, about 6–7 minutes. Remove kale to a colander and rinse with cool water to stop the cooking process. Gently squeeze out any water and chop the kale.

181. MAKE ADDING KALE TO YOUR DIET EASY

Cook up a big bunch of kale at one time and keep it on hand to use in any of the following ways:

- ▶ Add to soups just before serving
- ▶ Serve as a side vegetable with a dab of butter, salt, and pepper to taste
- ▶ Add to a vegetable stir-fry
- ▶ Roll up in a bean and rice burrito
- ▶ Top a pizza crust with it and add sautéed garlic, pine nuts, and feta cheese

182. BE A SNEAKY COOK

If you have difficulty getting the kids to eat kale, try puréeing cooked kale in their favorite tomato sauce and serving it over pasta. Just don't tell them what you did, and they'll never know.

183. CRUNCHY KALE IN MINUTES

This is a simple recipe that yields a crisp, chewy kale even your kids will enjoy snacking on. You can also slice up some collard greens or Swiss chard as a substitute for kale, or mix them all together for a tasty medley.

1. Preheat oven to 375°F.
2. Wash and trim 6 cups kale by pulling leaves off the tough stems or running a sharp knife down the length of the stem.
3. Place leaves in a medium-size bowl; toss with 1 tablespoon extra-virgin olive oil and 1 teaspoon garlic powder.
4. Roast 5 minutes; turn kale over and roast another 7–10 minutes, until kale turns brown and becomes paper thin and brittle.
5. Remove from oven and sprinkle with 1 teaspoon sea salt. Serve immediately.

GREEN TEA: SIP YOUR ANTIOXIDANTS

13

184. AMP UP YOUR ANTIOXIDANT POWER

The super-active constituents in green tea are a form of antioxidants called polyphenols (catechins) and flavonols. These antioxidants protect your body from the oxidative damage caused by free radicals, lowering your risk for diseases such as cancer, heart disease, suppressed immune function, and accelerated aging.

185. BOOST YOUR IMMUNE SYSTEM

Green tea significantly protects the immune system: White blood cell count was maintained more effectively in cancer patients consuming green tea during treatment.

186. FEND OFF WEIGHT GAIN

Green tea has been shown to prevent obesity in studies of mice receiving green tea in their diets. They showed a significant suppression of food intake, body-weight gain, and fat-tissue accumulation; lower levels of cholesterol and triglycerides; and a decrease in leptin levels in serum.

187. SAVE YOUR SKIN

Green tea may help prevent sunlight damage such as wrinkles and skin cancer.

188. KNOW THIS: WHO DRINKS WHAT

Most studies conducted on green and black teas, which are both from the Camellia sinensis plant, have yielded similar results. In 2006, Americans consumed well over 50 billion servings of tea, or over 2.25 billion gallons. About 83 percent of all tea consumed was black tea, 16 percent was green tea, and a small remaining amount was oolong tea.

189. WHY CAFFEINATED TEA MIGHT BE BETTER

Decaffeinated green tea is simply a more processed form of green tea, removing a certain amount of caffeine from the leaves. Due to this form of processing, green tea will have some of its nutrient content decreased. All green teas undergo some processing in the form of applied heat used to stop the natural oxidation process that occurs with freshly picked tea leaves. However, since this heat processing is minimal, the vast majority of nutrients are left intact.

190. BUY THIS DECAFFEINATED TEA

Your best and healthiest buy is water-decaffeinated or effervescence-decaffeinated green tea. According to one green-tea study, flavanol content varied 21.2–103.2 milligrams/grams for regular teas and 4.6–39.0 mg/grams for decaffeinated teas.

191. FIND YOUR FAVORITE FLAVOR

Bancha: A common leaf tea from the sencha plant, harvested as a second flush between the summer and autumn months. With larger leaves than the first-flush sencha, but with a weaker flavor.

Genmaicha: A light, delicious tea made up of a combination of maisha leaves and roasted brown rice.

Gyokuro: From a grade of green tea known as tencha. Gyokuro or Jade Dew refers to the pale green of the infusion. The flavor of the tea is influenced by the leaves being grown in the shade.

Hojicha: A roasted green tea; *hojicha* means "pan fried."

Kukicha: The roasted twigs of the tea tree, produced by harvesting one bud and three leaves.

Kabusecha: Another form of the sencha tea leaves, it means "covered tea," having been grown in the shade. It produces a lighter, more delicate flavor than regular sencha.

Matcha: This is the tea used in the Japanese tea ceremony. A high-quality powdered tea, it is also used to make green-tea ice cream and other forms of sweets.

Sencha: Probably one of the most common green teas brewed in Japan, made from leaves exposed directly to the sunlight, which may be why sencha means "broiled tea."

192. KNOW THIS TERM: TANNINS

Tannins in tea are large polyphenol molecules and form the bulk of the active compounds in green tea, while catechins make up nearly 90 percent of the tannins. Although there are no vitamin and mineral components to green tea, there are significant quantities of catechins present: Epicatechin (EC), Epigallocatechin (EGC), Epicatechin gallate (ECG), and Epigallocatechin gallate (EGCG). The most powerful of the catechins appears to be the EGCG, which accounts for 10–50 percent of the total catechin content; its antioxidant activity is about 25–100 times more potent than vitamins C and E.

193. BETTER THAN BROCCOLI

One cup of green tea may provide 10–40 mg of polyphenols and has antioxidant activity greater than a serving of broccoli, spinach, carrots, or strawberries.

194. CUT BACK ON CAFFEINE WITH GREEN TEA

The stimulant in green tea, called theine, was first discovered in 1827. Once it was shown to be identical to the caffeine in coffee, the word "theine" was replaced with the word "caffeine." Green tea contains a quarter of the amount of caffeine in coffee; 5 ounces of coffee has 80 milligrams of caffeine while green tea contains 20 milligrams.

195. AMP UP YOUR ALERT LEVEL AND STAY CALM

Theanine is an amino acid present almost exclusively in the tea plant. After drinking tea, theanine, which is present in green, black, and oolong varieties, is known

SUPERCHARGE WITH SUPERFOODS

to be absorbed by the small intestine and to cross the blood-brain barrier, where it affects the brain's neurotransmitters and increases alpha brainwave activity. This alpha brain rhythm is known to induce a calmer yet more alert state of mind. In other words, it induces a more calming, relaxed state, but one that allows the mind to focus and concentrate better at tasks. One cup of tea contains an average of 20–25 mg of theanine and the effect lasts about 3–4 hours.

196. KEEP YOUR MIND SHARP

Dr. Silvia Mandel and her colleagues at the Eve Topf Center for Neurodegenerative Diseases in Israel provided an amount of purified EGCG equal to about 2–4 cups of green tea per day to animals with induced Parkinsonism to evaluate how their symptoms improved or progressed. They found that when the animals were fed green-tea EGCG, the polyphenol appeared to prevent brain cells from dying and showed improvements in reducing compounds that led to lesions in the brains of animals with Alzheimer's disease. It also appears that the polyphenol may even rescue the neurons once they have been damaged and help them repair. The major question science is asking is whether these promising results are reproducible in humans.

197. BUY LOOSE TEA

With green tea, it is best to buy loose rather than in tea bags, as the leaves are uncrushed and usually of a higher quality. Cheap tea bags are often a combination of inferior-quality leaves, powdered tea, dust, and bits of branches.

198. PRESERVE THE FLAVOR

At home, place your teas in a container with a tight-fitting lid, as the tea leaves tend to absorb other aromas. Store in a dark, cool place and use within 6 months for optimal flavor.

199. QUICK TIP: STEEPING

Green-tea brewing time and temperature varies with individual teas. The hottest brewing temperatures for water are 180°F–190°F, and the longest steeping times 2–3 minutes. The coolest brewing temperatures are 140°F–150°F, and the shortest times about thirty seconds. For a medium-strength cup of Chinese green tea, simply pour boiling water over ½–1 teaspoon of tea and allow it to steep for 3–5 minutes. If the tea is left to steep too long in the hot water it will develop a strong, bitter taste. Loose tea needs a shorter steeping time than a tea bag, but if you steep for under 5 minutes you can't go wrong with the flavor.

200. REDUCE, REUSE, RECYCLE

You can use the same leaves to make a second and third infusion, which some people prefer to the first steeping.

201. COOL DOWN WITH A GREEN TEA CUCUMBER APPLE COOLER

This is a light, refreshing drink with multiple benefits from the cucumber, apple, and green tea. Sweeten to taste with stevia powder or sweetener of choice.

1. Wash 1 large cucumber, 1 large apple, and a handful of fresh parsley well.
2. Cut and section as appropriate to fit a juicer slot.
3. Juice all ingredients, add 1 cup chilled green tea, and sweeten to taste.
4. Serve immediately, while juice is still fresh and nutrient dense.

PUMPKIN SEEDS
HELP THE PROSTATE

202. PROMOTE PROSTATE HEALTH

Pumpkin seeds are effective in helping combat prostatic hypertrophy (BPH), an enlargement of the prostate gland that commonly affects men fifty years and older. BPH is caused by the hormone testosterone and its conversion product, dihydrotestosterone (DHT), overstimulating the prostate cells. Pumpkin-seed oil happens to contain certain ingredients found to interrupt the multiplication of prostate cells by testosterone and DHT.

203. BOOST BONE HEALTH

Pumpkin seeds are a good source of zinc, a trace element essential for the proper metabolism of nutrients. Although osteoporosis is usually associated with older women, it is commonly found in men who are deficient in zinc. A study of 400 men ranging in age from forty-five to ninety-two published in the *American Journal of Clinical Nutrition* found a clear correlation between not getting enough dietary zinc, low blood levels of the trace mineral, and osteoporosis in the hip and spine. Since zinc is also essential for prostate health, men should take in at least 15mg a day. A handful of pumpkin seeds, approximately ¼ cup, provides about 4mg of zinc.

204. QUICK TIP: STORAGE

Store your pumpkin seeds in an airtight container in the refrigerator or freezer to keep them fresh and edible for up to 2 months. The high oil content can begin to turn the seed rancid if exposed to air for too long.

205. TRY GREEN GOLD

Pumpkin-seed oil, which is known as green gold, has a pleasant and mildly rich flavor and should be used unheated in salad dressings, smoothies, or drizzled over steamed vegetables and greens. You can purchase it online or at your local natural-foods store. When purchasing pumpkin-seed oil, read the label to ensure the manufacturer has not diluted it with sunflower-seed oil. Extracting the oil from pumpkin seeds is a complicated and expensive process, reflected in the cost to you. Make sure the oil has been kept refrigerated both in the store and once you take it home.

206. EAT PUMPKIN FOR BETTER SKIN

Pumpkin seeds have been found to have anti-inflammatory benefits. So, eating pumpkin seeds may help reduce inflammatory symptoms of the skin such as eczema and psoriasis as well as arthritis conditions.

207. KEEP YOUR PUMPKIN SEEDS

The dark-green seed of the pumpkin has its own superpowers. This super seed contains a number of minerals, such as zinc, magnesium, manganese, iron, copper, and phosphorus, along with proteins, monounsaturated fat, and the omega fatty acids 3 and 6. Pumpkin seeds have been found to help prevent prostate cancer in men, protect against heart disease, and also have anti-inflammatory benefits.

208. USE YOUR PUMPKIN SEEDS

A handful of roasted seeds are nutritious and versatile. Here are ten suggestions to use them:

1. Toast and eat the seeds as a snack, with or without the shell.
2. Shelled seeds can be ground to make a Mexican mole sauce for chicken or fish.
3. Shelled, toasted seeds can be sprinkled over sautéed vegetables.
4. Sprinkle shelled and toasted seeds on soups and salads.
5. Grind raw, shelled seeds with fresh garlic, herbs, olive oil, and lemon juice for a salad dressing.
6. Replace nuts in your favorite cookie or granola recipe with shelled pumpkin seeds.
7. Raw or toasted shelled seeds can be added to hot or cold cereals.
8. Finely grind and add to rice and vegetables to make veggie burgers.
9. Use seeds to make toffee and brittle.
10. Ground or whole seeds can be added to yeast and quick breads.

209. TOAST YOUR PUMPKIN SEEDS

Here's how to toast unshelled seeds:

1. Give them a quick rinse with water then wipe off any excess pulp with a clean dishcloth. Spread the seeds out on a paper bag and leave overnight to dry out.
2. The next day, preheat your oven to 300°F. Lay out the seeds on a cookie sheet and season with a spray of olive oil, garlic powder, and sea salt. Place in the oven and bake 30 minutes, shaking from time to time, until golden brown.

Here's how to toast shelled seeds:

1. Heat a small, heavy skillet over medium-low heat and add 1 cup of raw, shelled pumpkin seeds.
2. Keep moving the seeds around the pan or shake the pan from time to time to evenly distribute the heat.
3. Within a few minutes, the seeds will begin to make a popping sound as they brown.
4. Reduce the heat to low and continue to toast until all the seeds have browned, then pour the seeds into a small bowl.
5. At this point, you can add a dash of soy sauce while the seeds are still hot and stir well. Be moderate; the heat from the seeds will dry the liquid, giving it a subtle flavor and salty taste.

210. COUNT IT AS A FRUIT

The pumpkin is really a fruit, even though it is used in many recipes as a vegetable. What makes pumpkins super is their low fat and sodium content, plus their orange coloring contains massive amounts of lutein and vitamin A in the form of beta-carotene. These antioxidants are powerful agents in preventing certain cancers. Pumpkin flesh is rich in potassium; fiber; vitamins C, E, and K; and many minerals.

211. MAKE THIS QUICK SNACK

A simple yet delicious snack you can make in just a few minutes. The heat from the toasted pumpkin seeds softens the raisins, creating a contrast in texture and a sweet-salty flavor.

1. Put raisins in a bowl large enough for the pumpkin seeds as well. Set aside. Have tamari ready at hand.
2. Heat a small, heavy skillet over medium-low heat; add pumpkin seeds.
3. Move seeds around pan to ensure each seed is toasted. As they brown they will make a sound like knuckles cracking.
4. Once seeds are brown and toasted, remove to a small bowl; add tamari. Mix well to coat seeds. The heat will dry the soy sauce. Be moderate—too much tamari will make the seeds soggy.
5. While seeds are still warm, add to raisin bowl; mix well. Set aside and allow to cool naturally. Store covered in a glass bowl in refrigerator.

NUTRIENT-RICH
MICROPLANTS

212. WHAT MAKES MICROPLANTS SUPER?

Microplants are an excellent source of two important phytochemicals: chlorophyll and lycopene. These super-powerful nutrients support your body's ability to detoxify heavy metals, pesticides, and other toxins and are loaded with nutrients to boost your immunity to disease.

213. KNOW THE MOST COMMON MICROPLANTS

Blue-green algae (cyanophyta): one of the first life forms. Presently available in loose powder or capsule form, blue-green algae contains beta-carotene and more nucleic acids than any plant or animal food. Actually, blue-green algae are composed of hundreds of types of algae, spirulina, aphanizomenon, and microcystis being a few.

Chlorella (chlorophyta): is a single-cell, freshwater green microalgae, and the first known form of plant life with a true nucleus. NASA considers it the ideal food for long-term space travel and colonization. It is useful for removing heavy metals, pesticides, and other toxic carcinogens from the body. It contains less protein and beta-carotene than spirulina, with twice the nucleic acid and chlorophyll. Its cleansing and rejuvenating properties fight aging, Alzheimer's disease, sciatica, palsy, seizures, multiple sclerosis, and general nervous-system issues.

Spirulina: a microscopic, spiral-shaped, blue-green algae native to shallow, brackish lakes. Spirulina provides more than 100 vitamins and minerals and is 60 percent digestible vegetable protein, with high concentrates of beta-carotene, antioxidants, B vitamins, iron, and chlorophyll. It's also a rare food source of GLA (gamma-linolenic acid), an essential fatty acid.

Wheat grass: a variety of grass similar to barley, oats, and rye, it is grown in fields across America, but the wheat grass referred to here is grown indoors in trays for approximately 10 days and then pressed into fresh juice. The 60-day-old field-grown grasses, available in dehydrated powder or tablets, are used primarily as nutritional supplements. Wheat-grass juice is made from sprouting wheat berries and is very high in chlorophyll. The chlorophyll helps cleanse the body, neutralize toxins, slow the aging process, and prevent cancer.

Barley grass: another green grass that is high in chlorophyll. The young green leaves of barley absorb crucial nutrients from the soil. Green barley leaves contain a multitude of enzymes, which supply the spark that starts the essential chemical reactions our bodies need to live.

214. DEODORIZE YOUR BREATH AND BODY ODOR

Chlorophyll helps deodorize breath and sweat, oxygenates the blood, strengthens body tissue, contributes to cell and tissue strength by aiding the blood in carrying oxygen, and promotes intestinal microflora. Chlorophyll in microplants nourishes, purifies, and suppresses inflammation in the body. Chlorella, spirulina, and blue-green algae contain more chlorophyll than any other foods—often double the amounts—depending on how and where they are grown. Chlorophyll can also be purchased in liquid form and taken as a supplement in a concentrated form.

215. KNOW THIS FUN FACT

African flamingos get their pink color from eating a super-rich diet that includes the pink-tinted microalgae known as spirulina. In the same way, if you were to drink excessive amounts of fresh carrot juice, your skin would take on an orange tint.

216. TURBOCHARGE YOUR IMMUNE SYSTEM

In 1979, Russian scientists published initial research on the immune-system-stimulating effects of lipopolysaccharides in spirulina on rabbits. Based on animal research, as little as 3 grams per day of spirulina may be effective for humans. It seems to turbocharge the immune system to seek out and destroy disease-causing microorganisms and cancer cells. Another study showed that spirulina boosted cells called macrophages—the first line of your body's defense—in chickens. The importance of these macrophage cells is their ability to communicate with T-cells to coordinate the fight against infections. Spirulina caused the cells to increase in number, become more active, and display more effective microbial killing.

217. BOOST YOUR CARDIOVASCULAR SYSTEM

People who regularly consume powdered organic barley-grass juice supplements could be providing a boost to their cardiovascular system, according to research published in the peer-reviewed scientific journal *Diabetes and Metabolism* (2002). In a clinical study, supplementation with barley grass reduced the levels of cholesterol and oxygen free radicals in the blood of Type 2 diabetics.

218. QUICK TIPS: BUYING AND STORING

Available in both capsule and powder form, look for a reputable manufacturer offering a blend that is certified organic. Store all your microplants in a cool, dry place or well sealed in the refrigerator. Once opened, they will keep for up to a month.

219. TRY MICROPLANTS IN THIS MORNING POWER GREEN SMOOTHIE

Feel free to vary the fruit using frozen strawberries, blueberries, or bananas. Add water to find the right consistency for your palate and adjust the sweetness to suit your taste. Combine 1 cup vanilla-flavored hemp-seed milk, ½ cup frozen blueberries, 1 tablespoon microplant powder of choice, 1 tablespoon flax-seed protein powder, 1 tablespoon hemp-seed protein powder, and your sweetener of choice (preferably stevia) in a blender; purée until smooth. Serve immediately, while chilled and fresh, chewing well to better release the enzymes needed to digest the proteins, carbohydrates, and fats.

220. COMBINE BROCCOLI WITH SEA VEGETABLES

The distinctive taste of broccoli and the mild-tasting arame sea vegetable are tied together in a cream sauce made from silken tofu. The perfect complement of flavors, East meets West in this mineral-rich vegetable dish. Silken tofu used in this way is the perfect substitute for heavy cream sauces loaded with heart-stopping saturated fat.

1. Cut the florets off 1 pound broccoli stems; cut into smaller florets and set aside.
2. Soak ¼ cup arame in hot water 10 minutes; drain and set aside.
3. Steam broccoli florets until tender; rinse under cold water and set aside.
4. In a large skillet, heat 1 tablespoon olive oil; add ½ onion chopped, ½ cup fresh basil leaves, and 2 cloves minced garlic and sauté until tender. Add broccoli and arame; stir well. Remove from heat.
5. In a blender or food processor, purée 1 (14-ounce) package silken tofu, 3 tablespoons mellow white miso, 2 green onions chopped, ½ fresh parsley, and juice of ½ lemon until creamy.
6. Pour tofu mixture over broccoli; mix well. Reheat gently if necessary, but do not boil.
7. Adjust seasonings and serve as a side dish.

221. EASILY USE ARAME IN OTHER DISHES

Soak arame in hot water until tender, about 10 minutes, then drain and toss with cooked grains, soba noodles, or a raw salad. High in calcium and other minerals, it is the most versatile of the sea vegetables and one everyone can enjoy.

222. GET A FEW VEGGIE SERVINGS IN ONE GLASS

There are quality green powder drinks that are a combination of all the listed microplants plus fruits, vegetables, sprouted grains, and probiotics. Makers of the leading green drinks claim that 1–2 tablespoons of this concentrated powder mixed in water will provide you with the equivalent of 5–6 servings of vegetables. Check the label for ingredients and nutritional breakdown.

OATS:
THE WONDER GRAIN

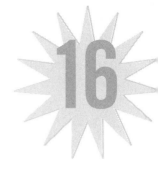

223. KNOW THIS TERM: WHOLE GRAIN

The whole grain consists of three parts. The synergy of these three components is what makes oats (and all other grains) so nourishing and healthy. This is the whole grain in its glory, before it has been stripped of its bran, endosperm, and germ and all their powerful nutrients, antioxidants, and phytonutrients to become a refined carbohydrate:

Oat bran: the soluble fiber-rich outer layer that contains B vitamins, minerals, protein, and other phytochemicals

Endosperm: the middle layer that contains carbohydrates, proteins, and a small amount of B vitamins

Germ: the nutrient-packed inner layer that contains B vitamins, vitamin E, and other phytochemicals

224. KNOW THIS FUN FACT

More oats are grown for animal feed than human consumption. Less than 5 percent of the oats grown are for humans.

225. GET MORE SOLUBLE FIBER

Oats contain more soluble fiber than any other grain. The soluble fiber in oats is known as beta-glucan. Beta-glucans are polysaccharides that occur in the outer layer or bran of cereal grains.

226. FEEL FULL ON LESS

Soluble fiber is the kind that dissolves in water, so the body turns it into a thick, viscous gel, which then moves very slowly through your body. As a result, your stomach stays fuller longer. What's more, it slows the absorption of glucose into the body, helping you avoid sugar highs and lows.

227. USE ROLLED OATS

It takes 10 minutes to cook regular rolled oats, while the thinner, quick-cooking rolled oats cook in 2–3 minutes. Instant rolled oats, which are the least nutritious, have already been cooked and dehydrated and just need boiling water to reconstitute them. For the highest nutritional value, use the regular rolled oats and save the instant kind for camping trips.

228. REMEMBER THIS COOL ANTIDOTE

In Samuel Johnson's dictionary, oats were defined as, "eaten by people in Scotland, but fit only for horses in England." A Scotsman's retort to this: "That's why England has such good horses, and Scotland has such fine men!"

229. DETERMINE WHICH OATS WORK BEST FOR YOU

There are a number of different ways that oats are processed for your cooking pleasure. The following is a description of the types of oats available, listed from the least to the most processed:

Whole-oat groats: minimally processed; the outer hull has been removed. Very nutritious and delicious, but need to be presoaked for 4–8 hours and cooked for a few hours. An alternative is to cook them overnight in a slow cooker.

Oat bran: the outer casing has been removed from the groat. The bran is particularly high in soluble fiber. Oat bran can be used as an addition to baking recipes or even raw in smoothies.

Steel-cut oats: also known as Irish oats, they have been chopped into small pieces, have a firmer texture than rolled oats, and are often preferred for hot oatmeal cereals.

Rolled oats: oat groats that have been steamed and flattened with huge rollers so that they cook quicker, in about 5–15 minutes.

Quick oats: groats that have been cut into several pieces before being steamed and rolled into thinner flakes, thus reducing the cooking time to 3–5 minutes. While they cook quicker, they lack the hearty texture and nutty flavor of the less-processed varieties.

Instant oats: groats have been chopped into small pieces, precooked, dried, and flattened with a big roller. They cook instantly with the addition of boiling water. This form of processing removes all traces of the original texture and rich flavor of the groats as well as many of the nutrients.

Oat flour: whole-oat groats have been ground into a powder, which may contain some gluten but not enough to make it rise like wheat flour. To make oat flour at home, place rolled oats in a blender or food processor and purée until desired consistency.

230. FIND HEALTHY FATS
The fats in oats are a healthy form, with a lipid breakdown of 21 percent saturated, 37 percent monounsaturated, and 43 percent polyunsaturated.

231. GET CANCER-FIGHTING NUTRIENTS
The germ and bran of oats contain a concentrated amount of phytonutrients including caffeic acid, a naturally occurring compound shown to be a carcinogen inhibitor, and ferulic acid, a potent antioxidant that is able to scavenge free radicals and protect against oxidative damage. It also seems to be able to inhibit the formation of certain cancer-promoting compounds.

232. LOWER YOUR CHOLESTEROL
Oats' cholesterol-lowering soluble fiber, beta-glucan, has been shown to lower total cholesterol by 8–23 percent in individuals with high cholesterol (above 220 mg/dl) when they consumed just 3 grams of soluble oat fiber per day—roughly the amount in a bowl of oatmeal. Given that each 1 percent drop in serum

cholesterol translates to a 2 percent decrease in the risk of developing heart disease, this is a significant effect.

233. EASE DRY AND ITCHY SKIN

Due to their anti-inflammatory properties, oats can be used for a skin-softening facial mask or wrapped in cheesecloth and placed in a hot tub of water to help ease dry and itchy skin. Try adding oat milk to your bath water. Begin by tying a handful of oatmeal into a piece of cheesecloth. While the water is running, hold the oatmeal under the faucet or let it hang while the water soaks through the cloth. With the tub full, place the oat bag in the water with you, squeezing it from time to time to release its milky properties. Use it to scrub your body and face so the juices can soften and cleanse your skin.

234. MAKE YOUR OWN MASK

To make an oatmeal honey mask: Take ½ cup of oatmeal; blend it to almost flour consistency. Place in a small bowl; add 1 tablespoon of honey and 1 beaten egg white. Mix well to form a paste and spread over clean face; relax 15–20 minutes. Remove the mask when done; rinse face well. This will leave skin smooth and soft.

235. THINK BEYOND OATMEAL

Rolled oats can be added to soups to thicken a purée and add a cream-like texture. Soak a few tablespoons of rolled oats in hot water for 5 minutes and add to your morning smoothie. Or replace bread crumbs with puréed oatmeal in meatloaf or burgers for added fiber.

236. UP YOUR OAT INTAKE WITH THESE ENERGY OAT BARS

In a large, heavy saucepan heat ¾ cup rice syrup on low until thin and runny, about 2 minutes. Add 1½ cups toasted almond (or peanut) butter and 1 teaspoon vanilla; stir well. Remove from heat; stir in ½ cup flax-seed meal, ⅓ cup unsweetened coconut, ½ cup rolled oats, ⅓ cup raisins, and ⅓ cup chopped walnuts; mix well. Spoon into an 8" × 8" casserole pan and spread; slice into 20 pieces. Cover and chill in the refrigerator or freezer.

237. COOK THIS FIBER-RICH DESSERT

Not too sweet but with plenty of chew, this combination of cholesterol-lowering oats and heart-healthy walnuts makes a great snack food. Take them to work to munch on your break and pack them into your kid's lunchbox. Either way, these two Superfoods provide calm, sustainable energy and nutrients for your brain.

1. Preheat oven to 375°F.
2. In a large bowl, mix 1½ cups rolled oats, ¾ cup spelt flour, ⅛ teaspoon sea salt, ½ cup chopped walnuts, ½ cup raisins, and 1 teaspoon cinnamon. Add 2 tablespoons coconut oil slowly, making sure to coat oats well with oil.
3. Slowly stir in ⅓ agave or maple syrup and ½ teaspoon vanilla extract. Add 1 cup cold water; mix until batter becomes thick.
4. Oil baking sheets with 1 teaspoon of coconut oil. Using a tablespoon, spoon batter onto oiled baking sheet.
5. Pat down each spoonful into patties about 2" across and ¼" thick and ½" apart. The cookies will not spread because there is no leavening agent.

6. Bake 25 minutes, or until golden brown.

7. Cool cookies slightly before removing from pan with a spatula. Cool completely before serving.

238. ADD VARIETY TO YOUR OATMEAL RAISIN CHEWIES

You can play with the ingredients, adding some of your or your children's favorite treats. Try adding ½ cup of carob chips or organic chocolate chips in place of the raisins or ¼ cup of unsweetened coconut flakes with some dried cranberries or dried cherries.

SWEET POTATOES:
RICH IN VITAMIN A

239. KNOW THE DIFFERENCE BETWEEN YAM AND SWEET POTATO

People are often confused about the difference between sweet potatoes and yams. The moist-fleshed, orange-colored root vegetable sold in American food stores and labeled a yam is actually a variety of sweet potato. It was the southerners who adopted the name "yam" to distinguish the darker-skinned orange sweet potato from the other varieties. There are about 400 varieties of sweet potato, varying in size, shape, and color. The flesh of the sweet potato can be white, yellow, or orange, with a thin outer skin in shades of white, yellow, orange, red, or purple. The shapes can vary from short and blocky with rounded ends to long and wide with tapered ends.

240. UP YOUR "A" INTAKE

For 90 calories per sweet potato, you get a huge amount of health-building nutrients. But that's not what makes it a Superfood: Sweet potatoes boast high amounts of beta-carotene—equal to that of carrots. That's four times the USRDA for beta-carotene when eaten with the skin on. In fact, one sweet potato has five times the recommended daily allowance of vitamin A, as well as being loaded with potassium. The potassium helps maintain fluid and electrolyte balance in the body's cells as well as normal heart function and blood pressure.

Sweet potatoes can be prepared as a cold salad, a rich stew, French fries, baked potato, or as a spread on focaccia bread. You can bake, sauté, steam, boil, fry, or roast sweet potatoes, and they always taste great.

241. GET MORE NUTRIENTS

The sweet potato ranked the highest in nutritional value with a score of 267, a full 184 points over its nearest competitor, the white potato, at 83 points, according to a 1992 study by the Center for Science in the Public Interest comparing the nutritional value of vegetables. The study was based on the following criteria: fiber content, complex carbohydrates, protein levels, vitamins A and C, iron, and calcium. In addition, the Nutrition Action Health Letter did a study rating fifty-eight vegetables for their USRDA for six important nutrients, similar to the ones listed above, but including folate, iron, and calcium. Once again, sweet potatoes topped the list with a score of 582 points, with its nearest competitor, the carrot, coming in at 434 points.

242. BOOST YOUR FIBER INTAKE

Cup for cup, sweet potatoes have been found to provide as much fiber as oatmeal.

243. BUY ORGANIC

Due to the possibility of pesticide residue on your sweet-potato skin, make sure to buy organic when possible or grow your own crop during the summer and autumn months.

244. SLOW ALZHEIMER'S

Consuming high levels of vitamin E delayed the progression of Alzheimer's disease by about seven months, suggests a study by Columbia University. Although present in a number of Superfoods, only sweet potatoes provide vitamin E without the fat and calories.

245. PREVENT DIABETES

With that sweet, delicious taste you might think otherwise, but sweet potatoes are considered a key food in preventing diabetes. It earned this designation in recent animal studies in which the sweet potato helped stabilize blood-sugar levels and lowered insulin resistance in test subjects. Some of its blood-sugar regulatory properties may come from the fact that sweet potatoes contain high concentrations of carotenoids. Research has suggested that physiological levels, as well as dietary intake, of carotenoids may be inversely associated with insulin resistance and high blood-sugar levels.

246. KNOW THIS TERM: INSULIN RESISTANCE

Insulin resistance is a condition caused when the body's cells don't respond to the hormone insulin. Under normal conditions, insulin acts as the key to unlock your cells in order for sugar to pass from the blood into each cell.

247. PROTECT YOUR LUNGS

For those who smoke or are frequently exposed to secondhand smoke, sweet potatoes, loaded with vitamin A, just may save your life. A common carcinogen in cigarette smoke—benzopyrene—induces vitamin-A deficiency, leading to emphysema. A diet rich in vitamin A can help counter this effect.

248. LOWER YOUR RISK FOR HEART ATTACK AND STROKE

Sweet potatoes are a good source of vitamin B6, which is needed to convert homocysteine, an interim product created during an important chemical process in cells (methylation) into other benign molecules. High homocysteine levels are associated with an increased risk of heart attack and stroke, but eating sweet potatoes can help in their prevention.

249. KEEP THEM TASTY

Avoid buying sweet potatoes displayed in the refrigerated section of the produce department, since cold temperature negatively alters their taste. The same applies to home storage, so don't store in the refrigerator or they will become dry and mealy when cooked.

250. COOK THIS NUTRIENT-RICH, LOW-CAL SOUP

Despite the sweet ingredients, this is a hearty and delicious soup. Increase the coconut milk to a full can if you want a richer coconut flavor. If you want to take the time, you can toast the cinnamon, garam masala, and cumin in a dry skillet over medium-high heat. Once they release their aroma, remove from the heat and add to the soup mixture.

1. Peel and chop 3 large sweet potatoes; rinse and drain 1 cup red lentils.
2. Combine sweet potatoes, lentils, 4 cups water, ½ teaspoon cinnamon powder, 2 teaspoons garam masala, and 1 teaspoon cumin powder in a large saucepan; bring to a boil.
3. Reduce heat; simmer until potatoes are tender.
4. Skim off any foam that forms on the surface while cooking.

5. When done, add ½ can coconut milk and sea salt to taste. Using a hand wand or blender, purée until smooth.

6. Serve topped with toasted pine nuts and a dollop of plain yogurt.

251. KNOW THESE INDIAN SPICES: GARAM MASALA

This combination of Indian spices is a traditional mix of cinnamon, roasted cumin, green or black cardamom, nutmeg, cloves, and mace. Garam masala helps warm the body and adds depth to a recipe. Make your own by buying the ingredients separately and grinding them in an electric coffee grinder or with a mortar and pestle.

WALNUTS PROVIDE ESSENTIAL FATTY ACIDS

18

252. REMEMBER MODERATION

In this chapter, you will learn about the walnut's tremendous nutritional benefits and how it can be used to raise the culinary standards of your menu plans. Just remember that more is not necessarily better, and eating too many walnuts can lead to considerable weight gain. After all, 1 cup (100 grams) provides 654 calories.

253. GET SOME OMEGA-3S

The walnut is a Superfood because it's the only nut that provides significant amounts of alpha-linolenic acid, one of the three omega-3 fatty acids. Because your body cannot produce this acid, you need to provide it daily from other sources. All it takes is seven walnuts to supply your daily need for these essential fatty acids.

254. HELP YOUR HEART

Just by having a serving of nuts five times a week you can significantly reduce your risk for heart disease. The high amount of unsaturated fat helps lower the

LDL (bad cholesterol) in your blood and increase HDL (good cholesterol). By eating walnuts, the omega-3 fatty acids are absorbed by the LDL particles, which in turn triggers the liver cells to remove this bad cholesterol from the blood. For every two walnut halves that you consume, the liver will lower the LDL particles by 1 percent. The many studies done on walnuts' ability to lower cholesterol levels have shown that for every 1 percent drop in LDL, there is a 2 percent decrease in coronary heart-disease risk.

255. OCCASIONALLY TRY WALNUT OIL IN PLACE OF OLIVE OIL

Walnut oil is more beneficial health-wise than olive oil because of the high amounts of omega-3 fatty acids. As one of the richest sources of polyunsaturated fat found in nature, walnut oil contains 60 percent linoleic acid and 12 percent alpha-linolenic acid. One tablespoon a day used in your salad dressing or drizzled over cooked vegetables provides you with the government-recommended daily dose of these heart-healthy fatty acids.

256. BOOST BRAIN FUNCTION

A walnut looks like a little brain, with a left and right hemisphere, upper cerebrums, and lower cerebellums. Even the wrinkles or folds on the nut are just like the neocortex. Research shows that walnuts help develop over three dozen neurotransmitters for brain function.

257. HEAL WITH WALNUTS

Every part of the walnut, with all its nutrients, has been used to benefit the human body in some way. The high B6 content helps alleviate premenstrual syndrome (PMS) in women. The vitamin E and zinc contents help keep skin

SUPERCHARGE WITH SUPERFOODS

smooth and supple, while the polyphenolic compounds help prevent allergic skin conditions such as eczema, especially in children.

258. EXTEND WALNUTS' SHELF LIFE

Once walnuts have been shelled they can go rancid quickly. When buying walnuts in bulk, keep them in tightly closed bags or jars and store in the refrigerator or freezer. Stored in this way, walnuts will keep for 6 months and sometimes up to a year. What's more, storing your walnuts in the freezer not only preserves their freshness, it keeps them out of reach for snacking purposes. Remove only the amount you will need for a day's use.

259. BEWARE OF RAW WALNUTS

Raw walnuts can harbor parasites, so it is better to soak them in a bath of 1 pint water to 15 drops of grapefruit-seed extract or roast them before eating. The grapefruit-seed extract destroys parasites and bacteria and the heat from roasting will help kill off the organisms as well.

260. WEAK APPETITE? TRY WALNUTS

Although walnuts are high in fat they are a good source of protein, which makes them a perfect food for individuals with weak appetites, the elderly, and those underweight due to illness. In these cases, and for those who cannot chew their food well, walnuts can be puréed in the blender with water, fruit, yogurt, and sweetener to make a delicious, healthy meal shake.

261. MAKE A BRAIN-BOOSTING SNACK

Walnuts are extremely versatile. Boost your brain power at snack time with a handful of roasted walnuts or coat them with melted butter and honey to make a sweet, crunchy treat. You could also combine walnuts with raisins, dried cranberries, pumpkin seeds, and peanuts.

262. MAKEOVER YOUR CREAM SAUCE

Make your cream sauce healthier with walnuts: purée them with water, maple syrup, and vanilla. Voilà—a rich cream sauce.

263. TRY THIS: ROASTED WALNUT TAPENADE

This is a versatile sauce that can be served over grilled chicken, meat, or lamb dishes. It will also serve well as a dip with vegetable crudités or thin slices of toasted bread.

1. Preheat oven to 350°F. Roast 1 cup walnut halves until lightly browned, about 8 minutes. Remove from oven and allow to cool.
2. Chop walnuts in a food processor using the pulsing action.
3. Add 4 teaspoons olive paste and 2 cloves garlic; continue to pulse for a chunky texture.
4. With the chute open, add ½ cup extra-virgin olive oil in a slow stream while you pulse ingredients.
5. Add ½ cup water, 2 teaspoons balsamic vinegar, and ½ teaspoon sea salt; continue to pulse until you have a smooth paste-like consistency.

264. HOW TO ROAST AND TOAST WALNUTS

To roast walnuts, preheat the oven to 350°F. Spread the walnuts out on a baking sheet and place them in the oven for about 8–10 minutes. Make sure to set an oven timer to remind you when they are done. To toast them, place them in a skillet with a little bit of oil and cook over medium-low heat, stirring often.

SUPERCHARGE WITH SUPERFOODS

265. SERVE GUESTS THIS SUPER-DUPER FRUIT DESSERT

When making the walnut cream, use just enough water to cover the walnuts. Let the blender run to ensure the sauce thickens and there are no lumps or pieces of nut remaining. This sauce is an excellent substitute for dairy whipped cream and can be served over cake such as strawberry shortcake.

1. Place ½ cup water, ½ teaspoon cinnamon, and ⅓ cup honey or agave syrup in a large saucepan; bring to a simmer.
2. Reduce heat to low, add 4 cored and chopped apples (skin intact); stir well and simmer for 1 minute.
3. Add 1 pint fresh blueberries; continue to cook until apples are just tender and blueberries have begun to release their juice, about 7–10 minutes.
4. Meanwhile, in a blender, combine 1 cup raw walnuts, 3 tablespoons maple syrup, 1 teaspoon vanilla extract, and enough water to cover walnuts; purée until thick and creamy.
5. Serve the fruit in a small bowl topped with the walnut cream.

266. OUT OF WALNUTS? USE THIS SUBSTITUTE

Cashews can be used in place of walnuts and make a rich and creamy sauce as well. For something more savory, leave out the sweetener and add some favorite herbs and sea salt. This makes a great protein-rich sauce to serve over grains and vegetables.

YOGURT REPLANTS YOUR INTESTINES

267. REPLANT YOUR LARGE INTESTINE

Live probiotic yogurt is a Superfood that has been around for over 4,000 years. Most beneficial of all is the abundance of live cultures found in yogurt that provide beneficial microflora where it is most needed—in your large intestine.

268. KNOW THIS TERM: PROBIOTICS

Probiotics are beneficial microflora—or good bacteria—found in the intestines.

269. EASE TUMMY TROUBLES

Yogurt is a high-protein food that can also be used medicinally to help with intestinal bloating, stomach disorders, and to relieve both constipation and diarrhea. When you have to take antibiotics (which can destroy the beneficial intestinal flora), it is best to eat freshly made yogurt to help replace the good bacteria.

270. PROTECT YOURSELF

Yogurt may help make the immune system more resilient, protect the intestinal tract, and increase your resistance to immune-related diseases such as cancer and infection, particularly gastrointestinal infection, according to a 2000 journal article in the *American Journal of Clinical Nutrition* published by Simin Nikbin Meydani, PhD. This is due in part to the live and active cultures, called *Lactobacillus casei* (LAC), found in yogurt.

271. LOOK FOR LACTOBACILLUS

Eating 1 cup of yogurt daily that contains the active *Lactobacillus acidophilus* has been shown to lower total cholesterol by more than 3 percent. The beneficial bacteria in yogurt, *Lactobacillus acidophilus* binds to cholesterol in the intestine and prevents it from being absorbed into the bloodstream. The reduction of blood cholesterol lowers the risk for heart disease. Thus, consuming probiotic yogurt may decrease your risk of heart disease by 7–10 percent. What's more, in a study of women volunteers, it was found that consuming 3 ounces of probiotic yogurt daily significantly lowered their LDL cholesterol while raising their HDL cholesterol because probiotic yogurt contains the beneficial bacteria *Lactobacillus casei*.

272. EAT YOGURT WHEN YOU'RE WATCHING YOUR WAISTLINE

A study published in the *International Journal of Obesity* indicates that including yogurt in your daily diet can help reduce body fat and minimize loss of muscle, good news for those on a weight-loss diet. It is thought that the calcium in yogurt reduces fat cells' ability to store fat, so your cells burn more and less is produced in the liver.

273. CUT BACK ON FAT

You can save 46 grams of fat per cup by using plain, low-fat yogurt in place of full-fat mayonnaise or sour cream, in equal amounts, for dips and dressings. The flavor and consistency will be similar and you will be doing your heart and hips a big favor.

274. MAKEOVER SOME OF YOUR CREAMY FAVORITES
Reduce the fat in your baked potato by replacing full-fat sour cream with low-fat creamy yogurt as a topping. Sprinkle with chives or chopped green onions, a dash of your favorite dried herb, and some salt and pepper to taste. Or use yogurt to replace heavy cream to thicken sauces. Add the yogurt at the end of the cooking process and remove from the heat, letting the sauce sit for a moment while the yogurt absorbs the flavors.

275. LACTOSE INTOLERANT? YOU CAN STILL GET THE HEALTH BENEFITS
Because the live organisms supply plenty of enzymatic action, fresh yogurt can be digested in approximately one hour, as compared to the three hours it can take to digest other milk products. If you have trouble digesting milk, you may find that fresh yogurt may be easier to digest and will actually aid in your digestion. For others who are lactose intolerant, avoid cow-milk yogurt and test your tolerance of goat- or sheep-milk yogurt instead.

276. IMPROVE YOUR ORAL HEALTH
Eating just 3.2 ounces (90 grams) of yogurt twice a day can help with bad breath. Yogurt lowers levels of hydrogen sulfide and other volatile sulfide compounds and helps eliminate tongue-coating bacteria and reduce dental plaque formation, cavities, and risk for gingivitis.

277. LOOK FOR THESE INGREDIENTS

Any yogurt that you eat should contain the live organisms *Lactobacillus bulgaricus* and *Streptococcus thermopholis*. These are the lactic-acid bacteria usually used to make yogurt in the United States. Also be sure to check the container's expiration date to ensure that it is still fresh.

278. MAKE YOUR OWN

You can make yogurt without an electric yogurt maker, but they are relatively inexpensive and make the whole process much easier. You can put it all together before going to bed at night and wake up to a batch of fresh yogurt in the morning.

The tools you will need to make your own yogurt include:

► Kitchen thermometer
► Yogurt maker with glass or ceramic cups
► 1–2 quarts organic cow or goat milk (you can use either low-fat, skim, or whole milk, but in general the higher the milk-fat level the creamier the yogurt will be)
► Small container plain, unsweetened yogurt with live cultures or a yogurt starter you can purchase from your local health-food store

Begin by heating the milk in a ceramic saucepan to about 170°F–180°F. Use your thermometer to check the temperature. This is done to kill any harmful bacteria that might be in the milk and to change the milk protein in a way that allows it to culture and firm up. Stir the milk continuously and watch carefully so the temperature does not exceed 180°F. You will need to sterilize your containers by pouring boiling water into them, letting them sit for 5 minutes, then discarding the hot water.

When the temperature in the milk reaches 170°F–180°F, turn off the burner and continue to stir it until it cools. Stirring the milk for another 2–3 minutes will prevent the milk from scorching the bottom of your pan. When the milk has cooled to 105°F–110°F, first mix the plain yogurt in its container to a smooth consistency then add it to the pot of warm milk. Stir it for a few minutes while the yogurt dissolves into the milk. This will allow the beneficial bacteria to spread throughout the milk and begin to grow. Now pour the inoculated milk into the sterilized containers and place the containers into the yogurt maker. Follow the maker's instructions for fermentation time, but normally it takes about 6 hours to set up. After about 6 hours, the yogurt should be firm. You can test it by gently turning the container to see if it keeps its shape.

There will be some whey liquid on the top that you can either pour off or just mix into the yogurt before you eat it. Cap each yogurt container and refrigerate. They will keep in the fridge for up to 2 weeks. You can use one of these live yogurts as a starter for your next batch, but you must do so within 5–7 days. You can also freeze a container of the fresh yogurt then let it thaw before inoculating your next batch of the sterilized milk.

279. AVOID ALUMINUM

Avoid using aluminum pans and bowls when working with yogurt, since its high acid content reacts negatively with aluminum. Best not to use aluminum for cooking at all, as it is known to leach into the food and cause possible health problems—one suspected, but not yet proven, problem is Alzheimer's disease.

280. OFFER DINNER GUESTS A HEALTHIER DESSERT

For the most health benefits, make sure to use organic yogurt containing live cultures of bacteria. Using organic for this delicious dessert can extend to the other ingredients as well.

1. Spoon yogurt into a small bowl. Add vanilla and maple syrup; mix well.
2. Lightly chop walnuts into large pieces; set aside.
3. In a long-stemmed parfait glass, begin with a layer of yogurt, then sliced peaches, and finally granola. Repeat layering to top of glass.
4. Sprinkle walnuts on top and serve chilled.

281. WHISK YOGURT, DO NOT BLEND

Mixing yogurt in a blender can cause it to break down and liquefy. Instead, either whisk it gently or fold the yogurt into the mixture when incorporating it into most recipes.

SUPERCHARGE WITH SUPERFOODS

FERMENTED FOODS: ESSENTIAL DIGESTIVE AIDS

282. KNOW WHAT MAKES FERMENTED FOODS SUPER

When foods are fermented, the bacteria, yeasts, or molds used in the process predigest the food, meaning they break down the carbohydrates, fats, and proteins to create probiotics, friendly, life-giving bacteria beneficial to the gastrointestinal system. Your body needs these super probiotics in order to function properly; they help keep your immune system strong and support your overall digestive health.

Fermented foods are enzyme rich and alive with microorganisms, known as friendly *microflora*. These colonize your intestines and work to keep the unfriendly intestinal organisms under control, such as yeast, parasites, viruses, and unfriendly bacteria. With a healthy, well-supported internal ecology, your immune system isn't overworked trying to keep the unfriendly organisms under control. Instead, it can take care of fighting infection and monitoring diseased cells in the body.

283. GET FAMILIAR WITH THE DIFFERENT FERMENTED VEGETABLES

There are a wide variety of fermented vegetables considered beneficial for healing the intestines and helping to maintain your health:

Cultured vegetables: A base of shredded cabbage and a few other grated vegetables, such as carrots and beets, cultured vegetables are packed tightly into an airtight ceramic, glass, or stainless steel container and left to ferment at room temperature for a week or more. The process pickles the vegetables, creating a more acidic environment for the friendly bacteria to reproduce.

Kimchi: A traditional Korean dish made by fermenting vegetables such as Chinese cabbage, ginger, garlic, and hot chili peppers. High in fiber yet low in calories, it provides 80 percent of the daily requirement of vitamin C and carotene. It is also rich in enzymes, vitamin A, thiamine (B1), riboflavin (B2), calcium, and iron and loaded with friendly lactobacilli bacterial cultures.

Pickles: Pickles contain large amounts of lactobacilli bacteria, important to the digestion of grains and vegetables. Scientific research has shown that these friendly bacteria survive the trip through the acidic juices of the stomach to the small intestine. In the small intestine they aid pancreatic enzymes in the transformation of *dextrin* (a carbohydrate found in grains) into simple sugars that can be readily used by the body. Other benefits of pickles relate to specific types, such as the alkalinizing properties of ume plum and the high niacin content of bran pickles. One property common to all pickles is high fiber, important to proper intestinal cleansing and function.

SUPERCHARGE WITH SUPERFOODS

Sauerkraut: Consists mostly of fermented green or red cabbage seasoned with herbs and salt. An excellent source of enzymes and *lactobacillus* bacteria.

Umeboshi plums: Japanese plums pickled in salt to create a powerful alkalinizing food. Umeboshi plums help neutralize fatigue, stimulate digestion, detoxify the body, and balance a sweet tooth. Taken the morning after, it is an effective hangover remedy.

284. GET FAMILIAR WITH OTHER FERMENTED FOODS

There are a wide variety of fermented foods considered beneficial for healing the intestines and maintaining health:

Vinegar: Specifically, apple cider vinegar. Rich in beneficial enzymes and used medicinally for centuries, apple cider vinegar helps strengthen the immune system, control weight, promote good digestion, balance blood pH levels, and remove toxic sludge from the body. Externally, it can be used to soothe irritated skin and relieve tired, sore muscles.

Coconut-water kefir: Made from the water of young, green coconuts and kefir starter.

Kefir: A fermented milk product similar to but considered more nutritious and medicinally beneficial than yogurt, kefir has more friendly bacteria, including *Lactobacillus caucasus*, *Leuconostoc*, *Acetobacter*, and *Streptococcus*. Because kefir needs to be made from kefir grains and not a powdered starter (often done commercially), it is best to make your own at home.

Kombucha: It is a colony of yeast and bacteria embedded in a pure cellulose "pancake" made up of beneficial microorganisms and usually fermented for thirty days. During this time, essential nutrients form, such as enzymes, probiotics, amino acids, antioxidants, and polyphenols.

Miso: Miso is a Japanese staple made from rice, soybeans, barley, or chickpeas. It is a fermented paste aged in wooden kegs for specific lengths of time. A light-colored miso is aged for 1–2 months, while the darker varieties are aged for up to two years. It is loaded with beneficial enzymes and traces of B12 and antioxidants.

Tempeh: A staple food in Indonesia, where it is traditionally prepared with soy beans or a certain variety of peanut fermented with the mold Rhizopus oligosporus. The culturing process binds the soybeans or nuts together with a thick, white myselium of new mold growth to form a cake. It has an earthy aroma, with a taste resembling a cross between mushrooms and fresh yeast.

285. FIND THEM IN PILL FORM

Lactobacillus acidophilus is a microflora commonly found in dairy products and fermented vegetables. *Lactobacillus planatarum* and *Lactobacillus brevis* are also helpful microflora found in fermented or cultured vegetables. These bacteria are destroyed when heated. Acidophilus is alive with microflora to aid your digestive system, so for a healthy gut and therefore a healthy body, take acidophilus capsules each morning on an empty stomach.

SUPERCHARGE WITH SUPERFOODS

286. LEARN WHY PROBIOTICS ARE BENEFICIAL:

Due to the prolific presence of pesticides, antibiotics, and preservatives in our foods, the beneficial microorganisms present in your body are being destroyed on a regular basis. These friendly microbes play a huge role in our digestive and immune systems' abilities to function properly. It is crucial that they are replenished from natural sources like kefir, yogurt, cultured vegetables, and apple cider vinegar.

287. GO RAW, AT LEAST OCCASIONALLY

Active enzymes—available in live and fermented foods—are generally only found in foods that have not been cooked, processed, or refined. They are the "spark plugs" for the body's cells because they put life back in your body.

288. BE FAMILIAR WITH THE TRACE NUTRIENTS

There are many trace nutrients in fermented foods. Here's a list of the many contributing organisms—in addition to probiotics and live active cultures—that make up fermented foods.

L-theanine: This is an amino acid that is known to promote relaxation and decrease mental and physical stress without inducing drowsiness.

Polyphenols: These are antioxidants that fight off the free radicals that stress the body and cause disease to occur.

Organic acids: These nutrients can help promote tissue and blood alkalinity and help normalize the natural process of homeostasis throughout the body.

Lactic acid: This acid helps maintain healthy digestive action (through the probiotic lactobacilli) and with glycogen production by the liver.

Acetic acid: This is an antiseptic and inhibitor of pathogenic bacteria.

Glucuronic acid: This acid is normally produced by a healthy liver, is a powerful detoxifier, and can be readily converted into glucosamines, the foundation of our skeletal system.

Usnic acid: This acid has selective antibiotic qualities that can partly deactivate viruses.

Oxalic acid: This acid encourages the intercellular production of energy and is a preservative.

Malic acid: This acid helps detoxify the liver.

Butyric acid: This acid protects human cellular membranes and combined with gluconic acid strengthens the walls of the gut in order to combat yeast infections such as *candida*.

Nucleic acids: These acids are like RNA and DNA that transmit information to the cells on how to perform correctly and regenerate.

289. KEEP THE CULTURES ALIVE

Store fermented foods in the refrigerator and use within 1 month of purchase to ensure the live cultures. However, if the fermented cabbage or kombucha

SUPERCHARGE WITH SUPERFOODS

drink loses its carbonated zing, do not be concerned; they may go a bit flat, but the probiotics are still alive and well.

290. TAKING ANTIBIOTICS? EAT FERMENTED FOODS

While the bad bacteria is being destroyed by the antibiotics, you are making sure the friendly bacteria is being repopulated in your intestines when you eat fermented foods containing live probiotics.

291. GO HOMEMADE!

Culturing your own vegetables is really your best option, even though it can take some time and effort. Most commercial products are created with taste in mind, not their medicinal effectiveness. In the case of yogurt, this means that commercial yogurt usually has a high lactose content and is loaded with sugar. Homemade yogurt can be made to eliminate a great deal of lactose and will be much fresher than anything you can buy in a store. If the taste isn't to your liking, you can add fresh fruit and or honey to sweeten it. Store-bought kefir has the same problems: You have no control over the lactose content in the end product. As for fermented vegetables such as sauerkraut, most commercial products have been pasteurized and do not contain live cultures.

The pasteurization process not only kills the beneficial bacteria, it may also destroy many of the enzymes and nutrients. Commercial sauerkraut may also contain a fair amount of unnatural preservatives. Fermenting your own foods at home is healthier, and less expensive.

292. MAKE YOUR OWN: GINGER PICKLES

Ginger is a wonderful root often used medicinally for digestive issues, nausea, and seasickness.

1. Peel and cut 4 pounds ginger root into very thin slices.
2. Using a wooden mallet or the flat side of a large knife, pound ginger slices to expel juices.
3. Place juices and pounded ginger into a glass jar; mix with 1 tablespoon salt and 1 cup distilled water.
4. Add ½ package yogurt starter; seal jar.
5. Let sit at room temperature 3–5 days, then store in refrigerator.

293. AVOID PLASTIC AND ALUMINUM

When fermenting foods avoid using a plastic or aluminum crock. This goes for your utensils, as well. Instead, be sure to use glass or enamel pottery specifically meant for making pickles and sauerkraut.

SUPERCHARGE WITH SUPERFOODS

EGGS FOR EYE HEALTH

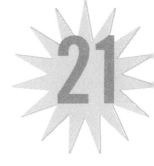

294. STOCK UP ON ESSENTIAL NUTRIENTS

For only 75 calories, one egg has 13 essential nutrients including protein, choline and folate—two essential nutrients that help with brain and memory development—and iron and zinc.

295. YOU CAN EAT EGGS

Twenty-four percent of Americans still avoid eggs for fear of dietary cholesterol, according to a recent survey by the Egg Nutrition Center, even though more than thirty years of research has concluded that healthy adults can enjoy eggs without significantly affecting their risk of heart disease. Unless your doctor advises otherwise, go ahead and enjoy eggs regularly. Remember that the American Heart Association still advises limiting cholesterol intake to less than 300 milligrams daily, and one large egg yolk has about 213 mg.

296. INCREASE YOUR VITAMIN D INTAKE

The yolk contains a higher proportion of the egg's vitamins than the white (except for niacin and riboflavin), and that includes vitamins B6 and B12, folic acid, pantothenic acid, thiamin, calcium, copper, iron, manganese, phosphorus, selenium, and zinc. All of the egg's vitamin D—as well as vitamins A, E, and K—are in the yolk. In fact, egg yolks are one of the few foods that contain vitamin D naturally.

297. EAT EGGS FOR THEIR CHOLINE CONTENT

Eggs are one of the best sources of choline, an essential nutrient that helps with brain and memory development. What's more, a higher consumption of dietary choline has been shown to lower plasma homocysteine levels. Why is this important? Plasma homocysteine is a known risk factor for cardiovascular disease, dementia, and Alzheimer's disease.

298. EAT TO BEAT BREAST CANCER

According to a study funded by the U.S. National Institutes of Health, more than 3,000 adult women with the highest intake of choline compared to women with the lowest intake lowered their risk of developing breast cancer by 24 percent.

299. BE NICE TO YOUR WALLET

Eggs persist as one of nature's best food bargains among high-quality proteins. At $1 per dozen large eggs, the consumer pays only 66.5 cents per pound for a high-quality protein. Compare that to a pound of fish, beef, or chicken.

300. EAT A HIGH-QUALITY AND GOOD SOURCE OF PROTEIN

What makes an egg a complete protein food is the fact that it has all nine of the essential amino acids. As a result, scientists often use egg protein as the standard against which they judge all other proteins (milk ranks second, fish third, beef fourth, and beans ninth). A large egg contains about 6 grams of protein—that's about 12 percent of the Daily Reference Value for protein.

301. SHARE THIS FUN FACT

Most eggs are laid between the hours of 7:00 A.M. and 11:00 A.M.

302. ADD EGGS TO YOUR WEIGHT-LOSS REGIMEN

Eating more protein-rich foods such as eggs helps preserve lean muscle tissue and increase fat loss during weight loss. Research has shown that when overweight and obese people ate a breakfast including eggs compared to those that ate bagels, the egg eaters felt satisfied longer and ate fewer calories over the course of the remainder of the day.

303. MUSCLE UP!

High-quality protein such as eggs may help healthy adults build muscle strength and prevent age-related muscle loss, suggests research published in a 2004 issue of the *Journal of the American College of Nutrition*.

304. PROTECT YOUR EYES

The yolk of an egg gets its color from yellow-orange plant pigments called lutein and zeaxanthin. It's actually the hens' diet, which includes yellow corn, alfalfa meal, corn-gluten meal, dried-algae meal, or marigold-petal meal that gives the yolk its color. Lutein and zeaxanthin are both carotenoids and have been shown to reduce the risks of cataracts and age-related macular degeneration, the leading cause of blindness in those sixty-five and older. The carotenoids, also commonly found in dark-green leafy vegetables, accumulate in the eye's lens and in the macular region of the retina. Scientists believe high levels of lutein and zeaxanthin in these areas may protect the eye from damage due to oxidation. What's more, research suggests that the egg yolk's fat content may make lutein and zeaxanthin more easily absorbed by the body compared to lutein and zeaxanthin from other sources.

305. BOOST YOUR OMEGA-3 INTAKE

At this point in the book you're well versed in the health benefits of omega-3 fatty acids. Omega-3s are commonly found in fish and seafood, but regular eggs also contain omega-3s (about 30 mg per egg). Up your omega-3 fatty acid intake with omega-3-enhanced eggs—one egg can have anywhere from 100mg to over 600mg per egg.

306. TRY EGG SUBSTITUTES

Most liquid egg products that you find at the grocery store are egg substitutes. Egg substitutes typically contain only egg white; the yolk has been replaced with other ingredients (e.g., nonfat milk, tofu, vegetable oil, emulsifiers, stabilizers, antioxidants, gum, artificial color, minerals and vitamins). Because each formula for replacing the yolk differs, you should check the nutrition and ingredient labels for total nutrient content.

307. FIND FREE-RANGE EGGS

Eggs labeled free range, according to the USDA, which regulates the term, means the hens are allowed access to the outdoors. Free-rang hens eat a grain-based diet and may also forage for wild plants and insects. From a nutrition standpoint, eating insects and other edible items may result in only a very small

SUPERCHARGE WITH SUPERFOODS

increase in the egg-protein content of free-range eggs and is considered insignificant. Lastly, higher production costs and lower volume per farm generally make free-range eggs more expensive.

308. MAINTAIN THE BENEFITS OF EGGS

To maintain eggs' nutritional quality, buy eggs only from refrigerated cases. Bring them home and refrigerate immediately (35°F–45°F or 3°C–7°C). Egg quality depreciates quickly at room temperature. Refrigerating your eggs at the proper temperature will allow you to keep them without quality loss for 3–5 weeks after you bring them home.

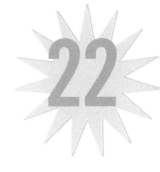

SLEEP BETTER
WITH SOUR CHERRIES

309. KNOW WHAT MAKES SOUR CHERRIES SUPER

Sour cherries get their bright-red color from anthocyanins, a powerful antioxidant linked to anti-inflammatory and antiaging properties. Sour cherries are a rich source of anthocyanins—boasting more than sweet cherries, raspberries, blackberries, and strawberries.

310. HOW TO REAP THEIR HEALTH BENEFITS

Tart cherries aren't the sweet kind you buy for snacking. They're the small, sour ones also known as pie cherries. Unless you like sour foods, tart cherries are likely too sour to eat on their own. But drinking the juice will give you the same benefits—and you can also add them to smoothies, quick breads, pancakes, and pies.

311. EASE JET LAG

It takes time for our body's internal time clock to adjust to an external time change, and as a result, frequent travelers sometimes turn to melatonin, a dietary supplement. Melatonin helps regulate biorhythm and natural sleep patterns. Turns out, cherries are one of the few food sources of melatonin. Scientists have found melatonin-rich tart cherries contain more of this powerful antioxidant than is normally produced by the body and thus eating cherries may be a natural way to fight jet lag.

312. DEFY AGING
Melatonin may do more than ease jet lag. A new study out of the University of Granada in Spain found that melatonin may play a role in delaying the effects of aging. Researchers discovered that melatonin neutralizes the oxidative and inflammation process caused by aging, indicating that melatonin can slow the aging process.

313. ALLEVIATE ARTHRITIS
Sour cherries have slowly grown a devoted fan base over the past few years. Arthritis sufferers believe eating sour cherries helps soothe their arthritic symptoms. Turns out, cherry consumption may in fact help relieve them: a recent University of Michigan study showed a cherry-enriched diet reduced inflammation markers in animals by up to 50 percent. Other studies point to the anthocyanins in cherries as being beneficial for inflammatory-related conditions like arthritis.

314. ADD THIS SUPERFOOD TO YOUR DAILY DIET
Tart cherries are available year round—dried, frozen, or in juice form. Here are a few ways to add them to your diet each day: make a trail mix using dried cherries, almonds, and whole-grain cereal; add dried cherries to tossed salad

or chicken salad; trade your raisins in oatmeal raisin cookies for dried cherries; or add frozen cherries, along with cherry juice and plain yogurt, to a smoothie.

315. BRIGHTEN UP BREAKFAST

It's easy to add tart cherries to your diet with these ideas: swap out the blueberries in your standard blueberry muffin recipe for fresh or frozen tart cherries; make a change from the typical berries that you top your cereal with to cherries; or add them to your favorite pancake recipe.

316. SIP IT LIKE A SPORTS DRINK

New research out of Oregon Health & Science University suggests that drinking cherry juice could help ease pain for people that run. The study showed that runners who drank tart cherry juice while training for a long-distance run reported less pain compared to those who ran but didn't drink the juice. What's more, runners who drank the cherry juice on race day reported a 2-point lower pain level upon finishing the race.

317. KNOW THIS TERM: ORAC

Oxygen Radical Absorbance Capacity (ORAC) units is a measure of antioxidant strength. In other words, a measure of how many free-oxygen radicals a specific food can absorb and deactivate. The more free radicals a food absorbs, the higher its ORAC score and the higher the ORAC score the better the food is at helping our bodies fight diseases.

318. GET MORE ANTIOXIDANTS

We should consume 3,000–5,000 ORAC units a day, according to some nutritionists, to have an impact on our health. Just one ounce of cherry juice concentrate supplies 3,622 ORAC units. That's nearly an entire day's recommendation. Want more? Cherry juice concentrate contains 12,800 ORAC units; dried cherries, 6,800; frozen, 2,033; and canned cherries, 1,700 ORAC units.

319. BOOST YOUR ENDURANCE

One antioxidant in cherries is quercetin. According to a recent study published in the *International Journal of Sports Nutrition and Exercise Metabolism*, you may be able to improve your exercise endurance by eating more cherries. The study found that quercetin (taken in supplement form) helped college students bike longer.

320. REMEMBER THIS FUN FACT

About 250 cherries are needed to make just one cherry pie. Each cherry tree has about 7,000 cherries; so, one tree can provide enough cherries for twenty-eight pies.

321. LEARN HOW TO PIT CHERRIES

Cherry pitters are available at most stores that sell kitchen equipment. If you have one, they're the easiest way to eliminate cherry pits. If you don't have a pitter, a paring knife will get the job done, just halve the cherry with your paring knife and then pry the pit out with the tip of a knife.

322. AMP UP THE ANTIOXIDANTS IN YOUR DESSERT

Make a quick sauce for desserts and ice cream: Heat fresh or frozen tart cherries with a little juice or water and sugar and thicken with cornstarch or arrowroot powder.

GRAPEFRUIT
FOR SMOOTHER SKIN

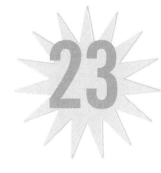

323. ADD GRAPEFRUIT TO YOUR DAILY DIET
Grapefruits are at their prime in the winter, but you can find them year round. They are an excellent source of vitamin C, fiber, vitamin A, potassium, folate, and vitamin B5.

324. REMEMBER THIS FUN FACT: HOW GRAPEFRUIT GOT ITS NAME
Many believe that the grapefruit is a natural hybrid of an orange and pummelo. Where they disagree is whether the orange was sweet or sour. Grapefruit actually got its name from how it grows on a tree—clustered like bunches of grapes.

325. TRY THE VARIOUS VARIETIES
White grapefruits are yellow skinned with yellow flesh and are bittersweet with a pleasant acidity. Red blush or ruby varieties have light-pink skin and deep-red flesh and are naturally sweeter and juicier. What's more, they boast lycopene, a phytochemical that may protect against prostate and breast cancers.

326. LOWER YOUR CHOLESTEROL

The soluble fiber in grapefruits may be helpful in lowering your cholesterol. Research shows that soluble fiber—also found in oats and beans—helps reduce LDL (bad) cholesterol levels.

327. KNOW WHICH ONE TO BUY

At the store, choose richly colored grapefruits with smooth, firm skin. Blemishes or scars suggest insect damage or improper handling during transportation. Pick fruits that yield only slightly to firm hand pressure and feel heavy for their size.

328. LOAD UP ON LYCOPENE

Red blush and ruby varieties of grapefruit contain lycopene. In fact, it's lycopene that gives them their color, which is why their white grapefruit counterparts do not have lycopene. Studies suggest that lycopene, also found in tomatoes and watermelon, protects against prostate and breast cancers as well as heart disease.

329. KEEP THEM FRESH FOR WEEKS

You can store grapefruits at room temperature 2–4 weeks. In the refrigerator, they can last 6–8 weeks.

330. PAIR GRAPEFRUIT WITH GREEN TEA

According to a study published in the *Asia Pacific Journal of Clinical Nutrition*, drinking green tea and eating lycopene-rich foods such as grapefruit together greatly lowered a man's risk of developing prostate cancer—more so than when either was consumed alone. Researchers suspect that consuming the two together offered a synergistic protective effect.

331. GET SMOOTHER SKIN

A cup of grapefruit sections contains more than 100 percent of the Recommended Daily Value for vitamin C. Eating vitamin C–rich foods such as grapefruits and oranges may help you lower your risk of age-related skin dryness and/or having wrinkled skin, according to recent research published in the *American Journal of Clinical Nutrition.*

332. DRESS UP YOUR GRAPEFRUIT

When you tire of digging into a grapefruit cut in half, spice up your grapefruit half by topping it with maple syrup or a dash of cinnamon or a dollop of yogurt. Cut it into segments to top your cereal or as a layer in a parfait.

333. STAY HYDRATED

Drinking water is the best way to stay hydrated, but water can get boring. Add natural flavor to your water with a slice of grapefruit. Even better, you can eat your water. At nearly 90 percent water content, eating a grapefruit can help you hydrate.

334. MOVE BEYOND JUST A GRAPEFRUIT

Slicing or peeling a fresh grapefruit makes a delicious breakfast or snack, but don't stop there! Mix grapefruit with avocado plus a little vinegar and honey for a yummy relish that can accompany chicken, fish, or pork. Or toss grapefruit segments with your favorite lettuce and a soft cheese for a satisfying side salad.

335. CHECK YOUR MEDICATIONS

Drinking grapefruit juice or eating grapefruits can enhance the effects of some medications and interfere with the effects of others. If you take prescription drugs, check with your doctor before you begin adding grapefruits to your diet.

336. TRY THIS HEALTHY DESSERT

Cut a grapefruit in half. On a heavy-rimmed baking sheet, place the cut side up. Adjust the oven rack so it's 6"–8" below the broiler element; preheat the broiler. Sprinkle grapefruit with raw sugar and broil it until lightly browned, about 2–4 minutes.

CRUCIFEROUS CABBAGE FOR STRONGER BONES

24

337. LEARN WHY THEY'RE SO SUPER

Cabbage is a member of the cruciferous vegetable family and offers compounds called indoles and isothiocyanates, which may help prevent cancer by amping up the production of enzymes that clear toxins from the body.

338. KNOW THIS VARIETY: COMMON

The common cabbage is also known as green cabbage. In general, it's round and firmly packed. The outer leaves are pale green and the interior leaves white.

339. TRY THIS VARIETY: NAPA

Also called celery cabbage, this variety is one of the milder ones, boasting a subtle cabbage taste and crisp texture.

340. GET MORE HEALTH BENEFITS WITH THIS VARIETY: RED

Red cabbage is similar to green or common cabbage in size, shape, texture, and density. As its name implies, it's reddish-purple in color. Anthocyanins, antioxidants associated with keeping the heart healthy and the brain functioning optimally, are what give red cabbage its color. It's the only variety of cabbage that boasts anthocyanins.

341. KEEP YOUR RED CABBAGE RED

To prevent your red cabbage from turning blue when you're cutting it, use a stainless-steel knife, as a carbon-steel knife will turn it blue. When using raw red cabbage in a salad or cooking it, add a little something acidic such as lemon juice or vinegar to maintain its reddish-purple color and keep it from turning blue.

342. QUICK TIP: BUYING

At the store or farmers' market, look for firmly packed and crisp leaves. Avoid those cabbages that have soft spots or cracks. Cabbage heads should feel heavy for their size.

343. KEEP IT COOL

In the refrigerator, you can keep cabbage for up to 2 weeks, especially if it's in the vegetable drawer. But did you know you can freeze it, too? You can! Cabbage can be stored in the freezer for up to 18 months.

344. CARE FOR YOUR CABBAGE

Here's what to do: Wash it thoroughly and remove the outer leaves; cut it into thin wedges or separate into leaves; blanch it in boiling water 2 minutes and then quickly transfer into ice water; drain off the excess moisture; put it into a container or freezer bag and then into the freezer.

SUPERCHARGE WITH SUPERFOODS

345. BUILD STRONG BONES

Vitamin K is abundant in cabbage: one cup of cabbage boasts 85 percent of your daily value. Recent research indicates that vitamin K helps reduce age-related bone loss. With age, cells that build bone become less active while those that break down bone keep working. Vitamin K fuels the proteins that rebuild bone and is also thought to positively affect calcium balance, a key mineral in bone metabolism.

346. DEFY AGING SKIN

Cabbage is a good source of vitamin C: one cup contains about 54 percent of your daily value. What does that mean for your skin? Data from the National Health and Nutrition Examination Survey I (NHANES I) suggests that middle-aged women who consume plenty of vitamin-C rich foods may have a lower risk of having wrinkled skin or age-related dryness.

347. ENTERTAIN YOUNG SCIENTISTS

This is a great (and safe) at-home science project for kids. Use red cabbage juice to gauge a pH level: add vinegar or lemon juice (an acid) and it will turn red; add baking soda (a base) and it will turn blue. Here's how to mix up red cabbage juice:

1. Grate the cabbage into small pieces and put them into a pot with water.
2. Boil the mixture 20–30 minutes, until the liquid turns a dark purplish color.
3. Pour the mixture through a strainer with a bowl below it to remove the cabbage, but preserve the juice.

348. EAT ON THE CHEAP

On average, cabbage costs less than $1 per pound—and that produces a salad that can serve a family of four, maybe more.

349. GROW YOUR OWN

Cabbage is very hardy and easy to grow. It originated along the Mediterranean seaboard, which is why it has thick and succulent leaves—to protect it from the sun and salt. Today, cabbage grows equally as well in temperatures just shy of freezing.

350. MAKE YOUR OWN SAUERKRAUT

Take a few tablespoons of the fermented cabbage with your meals to aid in digestion and the reimplantation of friendly microflora. Do not heat or cook the sauerkraut, which will only destroy the live organisms you need. To make your own, you can chop the cabbage in a food processor or grind it in a juicer that has a grinding attachment. Another way is to pound the cabbage with a wooden mallet to release the juices.

1. Chop 1 medium cabbage (red or green); set aside 5–6 whole leaves.
2. Place in a ceramic or glass crock or a stainless-steel container, filling to just ¾ full. (This leaves room for the fermentation to cause expansion.)
3. Add 2 tablespoons pickling or sea salt and 2 tablespoons picking herbs such as juniper berries; mix well.
4. Place whole leaves across top of cabbage to cover.
5. Gently press down on cabbage leaves to compress; place a plate on cabbage leaves and add a weight such as a few canned goods on top of plate.

SUPERCHARGE WITH SUPERFOODS

6. Place crock or bowl in a room with a temperature of 59°F–71°F for 1 week.

7. At the end of the week, remove weights and cabbage leaves as well as any moldy vegetables under the leaves.

8. Spoon sauerkraut into glass jars and place in refrigerator.

351. GO BEYOND SAUERKRAUT

Cabbage fuels Americans' obsession with coleslaw and sauerkraut. Did you know that Americans eat 387 million pounds of sauerkraut a year? They do! Move beyond these basic staples and try braising, simmering, or steaming it. You can also use the cabbage leaves as wrappers and fill them with sandwich ingredients or other stuffings.

ALMONDS: FEEL FULL ON LESS

25

352. LEARN WHY ALMONDS ARE SO SUPER

Over the past five years, almond consumption has gone up. That's no surprise, considering that ounce for ounce, almonds are the tree nut with the most protein, fiber, calcium, vitamin E, riboflavin, and niacin.

353. STICK TO A SINGLE SERVING

The recommended serving size for almonds is 1 ounce, about 23 almonds. Stick to the recommendation, as a single serving of almonds contains 160 calories and 14 grams of fat (1 gram saturated, 9 grams monounsaturated).

354. HOW TO GET THE PERFECT PORTION

Don't feel like counting out 23 almonds or lacking a food scale at home? Try these quick tips:

- Use an ice cream scoop
- Fill a shot glass
- Cover a 3" × 3" sticky note
- Pour your almonds into a ¼ cup measure

355. REDUCE INFLAMMATION

An ounce of almonds contains a generous amount of flavonoids, compounds that fight free radicals and reduce inflammation. What's surprising is that an ounce of almonds boasts as many, possibly more, flavonoids as a ½ cup serving of broccoli or a cup of green tea.

356. FIGHT FREE RADICALS

Free radicals can damage the body's cells, tissues, and even DNA, which is why researchers believe free radicals contribute to the development of chronic diseases such as heart disease and cancer. Almonds' vitamin E content (35 percent of your Recommended Daily Value) makes them antioxidant powerhouses and helps the body quell free radicals.

357. BETTER THAN BROCCOLI

Remember the ORAC score? It measures the total antioxidant potential of a food. The ORAC score for almonds is 4,454 umol TE/ 100grams—that's more than a baked sweet potato (2,115), avocados (1,193) and raw broccoli (1,362).

358. HELP YOUR HEART HEALTH

Yes, a 1-ounce serving of almonds contains 14 grams of fat, but only 1 gram contains so-called "bad" saturated fat and there's no cholesterol whatsoever. Plus, almonds contain heart-healthy nutrients including fiber, vitamin E, magnesium, copper, and phytonutrients. What's more, a handful of studies completed over the past two decades suggests that almonds may help maintain a healthy heart and contributed to the first FDA-qualified health claim for nuts. The claim states that, "scientific evidence suggests, but does not prove, that eating 1.5 ounces

144

per day of most nuts, such as almonds, as part of a diet low in saturated fat and cholesterol may reduce the risk of heart disease."

359. GET CREATIVE IN THE KITCHEN

Almonds are extremely versatile. Use whole almonds in their natural form, roasted, or flavored as a snack; top salads with slices or flakes; add slivers or halves to stir-fries and grain dishes; dice or chop and use as crusts for meats or in stuffing.

360. MAKE YOUR OWN ALMOND BUTTER

An easy way to add almonds to your diet is by swapping it out in place of peanut butter. No need to run out to the store either—you can make your own at home. Add whole almonds to a food processor and chop then blend in a little vegetable oil and salt until almost smooth. The end product will make a delicious topping to your favorite toast.

361. USE ALMONDS TO HELP YOU GET SKINNIER

In a study published in the *British Journal of Nutrition*, twenty healthy, overweight women added 300 calories of almonds to their diet for ten weeks. At the study's end, the almond-eating participants didn't gain weight. In other words, they naturally compensated for the additional calories from the almonds. What's more, researchers found that the fiber in the almonds blocked some of the fat calories from being absorbed.

362. FEEL FULLER LONGER

Almonds' fiber, healthy monounsaturated fats, and protein all help you feel full longer. A new study suggests that how much, or how little, you chew your almonds makes a difference, too. Published in the *American Journal of Clinical Nutrition*, researchers found that chewing almonds twenty-five or forty times—compared to just ten times—before swallowing increased the absorption of the healthy fats. Chewing forty times seemed to reap the greatest benefit: it suppressed hunger and elevated participants' feeling of fullness the most. Forty chews also resulted in elevated appetite-surpressing hormones.

363. KNOW WHERE YOUR ALMONDS COME FROM
California provides 80 percent of the world's almond supply. Almonds are California's largest tree nut crop and their top agricultural export.

364. REMEMBER THIS FUN FACT
The ancient Romans showered newlyweds with almonds as a fertility charm. Later, Italians began giving five sugar-coated Jordan almonds as wedding favors, each one symbolizing a quality of a happy marriage: health, wealth, happiness, fertility, and longevity.

365. EXTEND THEIR LIFE
You can maintain your almonds' quality for up to 2 years when stored appropriately. Keep them in the fridge so they stay cool and dry (the ideal condition is less than 40°F and less than 65 percent relative humidity). Also, prevent them from exposure to strong odors for prolonged periods, as they can absorb the odor of other materials.

SUPERFOOD RECIPES

QUICK APPLE CRISP

INGREDIENTS | SERVES 8
5 large red apples
½ cup raisins
½ cup apple juice
Juice of 1 lemon
¼ cup maple syrup
1 teaspoon cinnamon powder
2 cups raw oats (not instant)
½ cup walnuts
¼ teaspoon sea salt
1 teaspoon vanilla extract
⅓ cup vegetable oil
⅔ cup maple syrup

There is nothing like the taste of maple syrup, apples, and cinnamon heated together and baked—an American classic the whole family will enjoy. Serve warm with a scoop of vanilla ice cream or by itself. Delicious!

1. Preheat oven to 350°F.
2. Peel, core, and slice apples. Layer in a 9" × 12" baking pan with raisins.
3. In a small bowl, whisk together apple juice, lemon juice, ¼ cup maple syrup, and cinnamon; pour over apples.
4. To make topping, process oats in a food processor until almost flour consistency. Add walnuts and sea salt; pulse to lightly chop. Pour mixture into a large bowl.

SUPERCHARGE WITH SUPERFOODS

5. In a medium-size bowl, whisk together vanilla extract, oil, and ⅔ cup maple syrup. Pour mixture over oats; use a wooden spoon to combine. You may need to use your hands to mix well enough to coat oats and walnuts.

6. When done, spoon mixture over top of apples. Bake 30 minutes, or until apples are tender and topping is a golden brown.

7. Allow to cool slightly before serving.

440 calories | 16g fat | 74g carbohydrates | 5g protein | 44g sugars | 7g fiber

---

MAPLE SYRUP

Maple syrup is made from the sap of the sugar, black or red maple tree. The tree is first tapped (pierced), which allows the sap to run out freely. The clear, tasteless sap is then boiled down to evaporate the water, giving it the characteristic maple flavor and amber color, with a sugar content of 60 percent.

CREPES WITH APPLE BLUEBERRY FILLING

INGREDIENTS | SERVES 8

CREPES
4 eggs
1 cup soy or rice milk
½ cup water
½ teaspoon sea salt
1 cup spelt flour
3 tablespoons melted ghee

APPLE BLUEBERRY FILLING
1 apple
1 pear
Pinch of stevia powder
1 cup water
2 cups blueberries
1 tablespoon kudzu powder
2 tablespoons xylitol

This crepe recipe can be used with roasted vegetables and walnut parsley sauce or with other cooked vegetables and topped with grated Romano cheese.

CREPE:
1. Combine all crepe ingredients in a blender; purée until smooth. Scrape sides and purée until everything is combined. Place in fridge 2 hours, or overnight.

SUPERCHARGE WITH SUPERFOODS

2. Heat a crepe pan; spray with oil. When hot, pour ¼ cup batter onto a 10" pan (2 tablespoons for a 7" pan); swirl around to cover bottom. Cook until browned on bottom, about 1 minute.

3. Loosen crepe with a spatula or knife; flip with your fingers. Cook second side about 30 seconds.

4. Stack crepes to keep them warm; cover with a clean cloth towel.

FILLING:

1. Peel and core apple and pear; slice and place in a heavy saucepan with sweetener and ½ cup water.

2. Add blueberries; bring mixture to a simmer. Cook until fruit is tender, about 10 minutes.

3. Dissolve kudzu powder in remaining water; add to fruit while cooking. Stir until liquid thickens. Remove from heat and set aside.

4. Lay out a crepe on a plate; spoon fruit mixture onto one half of crepe. Fold crepe over; sprinkle top with xylitol and/or cinnamon.

180 calories | 8g fat | 22g carbohydrates | 6g protein | 7g sugars | 4g fiber

HERBAL SWEETENER

Stevia is an herbal sweetener used by diabetics and dieters and actually helps balance blood-sugar levels The herb *stevia rebaudiana* is a member of the South American daisy family. It is 300 times sweeter than regular sugar, contains no calories, and is heat stable. Finally, a great alternative to refined and artificial sweeteners!

BROCCOLI AND TOMATOES IN ANCHOVY SAUCE

INGREDIENTS | SERVES 4

⅓ cup extra-virgin olive oil

3 cloves garlic

6 anchovy fillets or 2 tablespoons anchovy paste

½ cup fresh parsley, stems removed

1 pound broccoli florets

2 large ripe tomatoes

½ cup grated Romano cheese

Sea salt to taste

The broccoli and tomatoes can be tossed with the sauce and served as a side dish, or the whole thing can be combined with cooked angel-hair pasta and served with a fresh green salad and a hunk of country whole-grain bread.

1. In a mortar and pestle or food processor, combine oil, garlic, anchovies, and parsley; process to a loose paste. Add more oil as needed for consistency.
2. Steam or simmer broccoli until just tender. Remove from the heat; place in a medium-size bowl.
3. Quarter and chop tomatoes; add to broccoli.
4. Spoon anchovy sauce into broccoli and tomatoes; toss gently to coat.
5. Sprinkle with Romano cheese, add salt as desired, and serve.

260 calories | 21g fat | 12g carbohydrates | 8g protein | 2g sugars | 5g fiber

SUPERCHARGE WITH SUPERFOODS

QUINOA WITH SAUTÉED GARLIC

INGREDIENTS | SERVES 4–6

1 cup quinoa
2 cups water or vegetable stock
½ teaspoon sea salt
½ medium onion
6 cloves garlic
¼ cup extra-virgin olive oil

This is the type of recipe that can become a staple in your kitchen.
Quick, easy, and a very delicious way to prepare any type of grain.
Of course, anything tastes great tossed with olive oil and garlic!

1. Place quinoa in a metal strainer; rinse well under running water. Drain; add to a heavy saucepan with water or stock and sea salt.
2. Chop onion; add to quinoa.
3. Cover and bring to a boil over medium-high heat; reduce heat and simmer until all water has been absorbed, about 15–20 minutes.
4. Meanwhile, slice garlic lengthwise along clove; set aside.
5. Heat oil in a small skillet; sauté garlic until just crisp but not yet brown. Remove from heat.
6. When quinoa is done, pour garlic and oil over quinoa; toss gently. Serve as a side dish or top with stir-fried beans and vegetables for a main dish.

200 calories | 11g fat | 22g carbohydrates | 4g protein | 0g sugars | 2g fiber

QUINOA BLACK BEAN SALAD

INGREDIENTS | SERVES 8

1 cup quinoa
2 cups water
½ teaspoon salt
1 carrot
2 green onions
⅓ cup pumpkin seeds
½ cup parsley leaves
1 (14-ounce) can of black beans
Juice of 1 lemon
1 clove minced garlic
2 tablespoons apple cider vinegar
3 tablespoons extra virgin olive oil
½ teaspoon salt

For grain salads, the longer it marinates the better the flavors are absorbed by the ingredients. Make it the night before and take some to work for lunch the next day. Bring this salad along for a potluck meal and watch how your friends enjoy something new and delicious.

1. In a medium saucepan, combine quinoa, water, and ½ teaspoon sea salt. Cover, bring to a boil, reduce heat to low, and simmer until all water is absorbed, about 20 minutes. When done, spoon into a large bowl and allow to cool.

SUPERCHARGE WITH SUPERFOODS

2. Meanwhile, grate carrots, slice onions, toast pumpkin seeds, mince parsley, and rinse canned beans.

3. When quinoa is cool, add carrots, green onions, pumpkin seeds, black beans, and parsley; mix well.

4. In a small bowl, whisk together lemon, garlic, vinegar, oil, and salt.

5. Add vinaigrette; mix completely and allow to marinate a few minutes before serving.

190 calories | 7g fat | 26g carbohydrates | 6g protein | 1g sugars | 5g fiber

QUINOA PARSLEY TABBOULEH

INGREDIENTS | SERVES 6

1 cup quinoa
2 cups water or vegetable broth
½ teaspoon sea salt
1 cup fresh parsley
3 green onions
1 cup plum tomatoes
1 clove garlic
¼ cup extra-virgin olive oil
Juice of 1 lemon
Sea salt to taste

Make sure to seed the tomatoes for easier digestion, but also to prevent excess liquid from making your tabbouleh soggy.

1. In a heavy saucepan, combine quinoa, water, and sea salt; bring to a boil.
2. Reduce heat and simmer until all water is absorbed, about 15–20 minutes.
3. When quinoa is done, spoon into a large bowl and allow to cool.
4. While quinoa cools, mince parsley and green onion; set aside.
5. Halve tomatoes lengthwise; scoop out seeds into a measuring cup or small bowl.
6. Chop tomatoes into small pieces; add to parsley and green onions.
7. Press and mince garlic; whisk together in a small bowl with oil, lemon juice, and sea salt.

SUPERCHARGE WITH SUPERFOODS

8. Strain and discard tomato seeds; add tomato liquid to lemon dressing.
9. Add parsley, green onion, and tomatoes to quinoa; toss well.
10. Add lemon dressing; mix well to combine all ingredients. Adjust seasonings with salt if needed.

210 calories | 11g fat | 23g carbohydrates | 4g protein | 2g sugars | 2g fiber

QUINOA BREAKFAST CONGEE

INGREDIENTS | SERVES 4

¼ cup hijiki
½ onion
½ cup quinoa
½ cup brown rice
½ teaspoon sea salt
5 cups water
¼ cup toasted pumpkin seeds

Congee is a porridge traditionally made with rice and is primarily eaten as a breakfast food. It can be fed to individuals who are unable to chew due to illness or poor digestion. Congee takes a long time to cook, so it can be made in a rice cooker or slow cooker overnight.

1. Soak hijiki in hot water 10 minutes; drain and set aside.
2. Chop onion; set aside.
3. Before going to bed, plug in 1.5-quart slow cooker and add quinoa, rice, hijiki, onion, sea salt, and water. Set temperature on low; cook overnight. (You can also use a rice cooker if it has a setting for congee, as some do.)
4. In the morning, toast pumpkin seeds in a dry skillet; set aside.
5. Stir congee; spoon into individual serving bowls. Top with pumpkin seeds and serve with cooked greens such as kale, spinach, or broccoli.

193 calories | 2.5g fat | 37g carbohydrates | 5g protein | 1g sugars | 3g fiber

WHEAT-FREE BROWNIES

INGREDIENTS | SERVES 8, 2" × 4" BARS

1½ cups brown rice flour

1 cup unsweetened cocoa powder

¼ teaspoon sea salt

1 (10-ounce) package soft silken tofu

1 teaspoon orange extract

1 teaspoon vanilla extract

½ cup barley malt

½ cup maple syrup

1 cup low-fat soy or rice milk

⅔ cup walnuts

1. Preheat oven to 350°F.
2. In a medium-size bowl, combine flour, cocoa, and salt.
3. In a blender, purée tofu, orange extract, vanilla extract, barley malt, maple syrup, and milk.
4. Stir tofu mixture into flour mixture; add walnuts and mix well.
5. Pour into a lightly oiled 8" × 8" baking dish; bake 30 minutes.

320 calories | 10g fat | 54g carbohydrates | 9g protein | 13g sugars | 6g fiber

DARK CHOCOLATE

When a recipe calls for chocolate, use dark chocolate (usually less sugar) or even better, cocoa powder. To substitute 1 ounce of unsweetened chocolate, use 3 tablespoons dry cocoa + 2 tablespoons sugar + 1 tablespoon mild-flavored vegetable oil.

WILD RICE MINT SALAD WITH ARAME

INGREDIENTS | SERVES 8

½ cup pine nuts, toasted
½ cup arame, cooked
3 cups cooked long-grain brown rice (1½ cups uncooked)
1 cup cooked wild rice (½ cup uncooked)
2 green onions, chopped
½ cup parsley, minced
½ cup fresh mint, minced
1 teaspoon fresh thyme
2 tablespoons red wine vinegar
1 teaspoon ume plum vinegar
3 tablespoons extra-virgin olive oil

This is the perfect way to introduce arame into your diet. The recipe is loaded with flavor, complemented by arame's light salty taste. Serve with cold poached salmon topped with aioli mayonnaise and a fresh green salad.

1. Toast the pine nuts in a heavy nonoiled skillet, shaking to evenly brown on all sides. Set aside in a bowl.
2. Soak arame in water 10 minutes. Drain; place in a small saucepan. Cover with water; bring to a boil and simmer 10 minutes. Drain; set aside to cool.
3. In a large bowl, combine brown rice, wild rice, onion, arame, parsley, mint, and thyme; mix well.

4. In a separate bowl, mix together red wine vinegar, ume vinegar, and oil.

5. Pour dressing over rice mixture; toss well. Add pine nuts and serve.

210 calories | 12g fat | 23g carbohydrates | 4g protein | 1g sugars | 2g fiber

WILD RICE

A member of the grass family of plants, native to North America, and a staple in the diet of early Native Americans, wild rice is a large seed grown primarily in the Great Lakes region. A nutritional grain higher in protein than cultivated brown rice and low in fat, its mineral content is high in potassium and phosphorus.

ROASTED GARLIC AIOLI MAYONNAISE

INGREDIENTS | MAKES I CUP

I head garlic
¾ cup extra-virgin olive oil
I organic egg
I tablespoon fresh lemon juice
I tablespoon raw apple cider vinegar
Pinch sea salt

To save time or when you don't have a blender, you can use I cup of a good-quality store-bought mayonnaise in place of making it from scratch. Add dried herbs of your choice for extra flavor. Serve over vegetables, grilled meats, fish, or swirled into a thick purée of hot lentil soup.

1. Preheat oven to 375°F.
2. Wrap garlic in aluminum foil; bake 20 minutes.
3. Allow to cool, remove foil, and slice across flat end of head.
4. Squeeze softened cloves out end into a small bowl; set aside.
5. Pour ¼ cup oil into a blender with egg, lemon juice, vinegar, and salt.
6. Turn on blender; pour remaining oil into mixture in a slow stream. Mayonnaise will thicken as you pour the oil.
7. Add roasted garlic to mayonnaise; pulse to combine. Run blender additional 30 seconds after garlic has been added.
8. Keep mixture refrigerated in a glass container 5–7 days.

1680 calories | 173g fat | 22g carbohydrates | 10g protein | 1g sugars | 1g fiber

SUPERCHARGE WITH SUPERFOODS

CREAMY GARLIC SOUP

INGREDIENTS
6 cups chicken or vegetable stock
4 dried shitake mushrooms
4 heads garlic
1 teaspoon sea salt
14 ounces silken tofu
6 teaspoons extra-virgin olive oil
¼ cup minced parsley
¼ cup toasted pine nuts

The shiitake mushrooms add a distinctive flavor to the stock. Once they have soaked you can slice them and use them later in a stir-fry or morning omelet.

1. Preheat oven to 375°F.
2. In a large saucepan, add stock and mushrooms; simmer gently.
3. Wrap garlic in aluminum foil; bake 20 minutes, or until tender.
4. Remove garlic from oven; allow to cool. Remove aluminum foil; slice off flat end of garlic head. Squeeze softened cloves into a bowl; set aside.
5. In a blender, purée roasted garlic, salt, silken tofu, and 2 cups stock.
6. Remove mushrooms from stock and set aside to use at another time. Add puréed tofu mixture to stock; heat just until warmed through.
7. Ladle soup into individual bowls; drizzle a teaspoon of olive oil along surface. Top with minced parsley and toasted pine nuts.

270 calories | 11g fat | 36g carbohydrates | 10g protein | 3g sugars | 3g fiber

AVOCADO PLUM SALAD

INGREDIENTS | SERVES 8
Juice of 1 lemon
1 teaspoon ume plum vinegar
1 tablespoon agave syrup
2 tablespoons extra-virgin olive oil
2 cups red radish, quartered
½ cup toasted walnuts, chopped
2 cups baby plums, pitted and halved
2 ripe Haas avocados, diced

Red grapes can be substituted for the plums if desired. Try not to over stir the ingredients or the avocado will break down and lose its shape.

1. In a medium-size bowl, whisk together lemon juice, vinegar, agave, and olive oil.
2. Add radish, walnuts, and baby plums to dressing; toss to cover.
3. Add avocado; toss gently to cover with dressing.
4. Place in refrigerator for 10 minutes to chill before serving.

190 calories | 16g fat | 12g carbohydrates | 3g protein | 5g sugars | 5g fiber

---

UME PLUM VINEGAR
Cherry-pink in color, ume plum vinegar is made from Japanese pickled umeboshi plums. It has a salty, sour flavor with light citrus undertones. It is a great substitute for salt in salad dressings and sauces.

AVOCADO REUBEN SANDWICHES

INGREDIENTS | SERVES 4

1 (10-ounce) package soy tempeh
8 slices whole-grain bread
2 tablespoons olive oil
8 tablespoons Thousand Island dressing, divided
1½ cups sauerkraut
1 ripe avocado
4 slices Monterey jack cheese

*Commercial Thousand Island dressing can be used, but for a taste treat make
your own by combining 1 cup of mayonnaise with ½ cup of your favorite salsa.
This recipe works well as a topping for turkey or veggie burgers as well.*

1. Cut block of tempeh in half, then cut in half crosswise, making 4 thin slabs.
2. Lightly toast bread.
3. Heat oil in a heavy skillet; brown tempeh slabs on both sides.
4. Arrange 4 pieces of bread on separate plates; spread each with 1 tablespoon dressing. Top each slice with a slab of tempeh, spoonful of sauerkraut, a few slices of avocado, and a slice of cheese.
5. Place sandwich half under broiler to melt cheese.
6. Spread another tablespoon of dressing on second piece of bread; lay it on
top of cheese.
7. Slice each sandwich on diagonal and serve immediately.

660 calories | 41g fat | 52g carbohydrates | 26g protein | 12g sugars | 14g fiber

SALMON CAKES WITH MANGO SALSA

INGREDIENTS | SERVES 4

1 (14-ounce) can wild Alaskan salmon
¼ cup minced chives
1 large egg, beaten
1 cup almond or pecan flour
Sea salt to taste
1 ripe mango
½ sweet Vidalia onion
½ red pepper
3" piece ginger root
Juice of 1 lemon

If you cannot find almond or pecan meal, you can make your own by grinding a cup of raw almonds or pecans in a food processor until a flour consistency is achieved. Be careful not to run it so long it becomes an oily paste.

1. Preheat oven to 350°F.
2. In a medium bowl, combine salmon, chives, beaten egg, nut flour, and sea salt.
3. Mix well; form into 4 patties.
4. Place on a well-oiled baking sheet; bake 15–20 minutes, or cook in an oiled skillet, browning on both sides.
5. To make the salsa, peel and chop mango into small pieces; place in a medium-size bowl.
6. Mince red pepper and onion; add to bowl.

SUPERCHARGE WITH SUPERFOODS

7. Peel and grate ginger, extracting juice by pressing the fiber against the side of a shallow dish; pour juice into bowl with mango mixture.
8. Juice the lemon; add to mango mixture and mix well.
9. Cover and refrigerate until ready to serve. For a hotter, spicier version, add a fresh, minced jalapeño pepper.

260 calories | 8g fat | 18g carbohydrates | 30g protein | 11g sugars | 4g fiber

GRILLED SALMON AND SALSA

A beautiful fillet of grilled salmon would benefit from a few tablespoons of mango or tomato salsa. The juices will enrich the dry meat and the sweet-sour taste will only complement the smoky flavor of the fish. Serve alongside some steamed broccoli tossed with garlic sautéed in olive oil and a salad of cooked kale and walnuts. A true Superfoods meal.

SUMMER SALMON SALAD

INGREDIENTS | SERVES 4
1 large beefsteak tomato
½ cup fresh parsley
⅓ cup fresh basil
1 shallot
12 walnut halves
2 slices thick sour dough bread
1 (10-ounce) can wild sockeye salmon
Juice of ½ lemon
2 tablespoons extra-virgin olive oil
½ cup orange juice
1 teaspoon orange zest
½ teaspoon honey
2 tablespoons white-wine vinegar
½ teaspoon ume plum vinegar
1 clove minced garlic
½ cup grated Romano cheese

*This salad is reminiscent of a Tuscan bread salad and needs
a little time to marinate before serving. Allow the bread to
soak up some of the dressing but not get too soggy.*

1. Slice tomato into bite-size pieces; place in a medium-size ceramic bowl.
2. Mince parsley and basil until very fine; add to tomatoes.
3. Slice shallot into thin half moons; add to tomatoes.

4. Break walnuts into pieces with your hands; add to tomatoes.

5. Lightly toast bread; slice into bite-size cubes and add to tomatoes.

6. Open can of salmon and separate skin and visible bones; place in a bowl and squeeze some lemon over salmon. Set aside.

7. In a small bowl, whisk together oil, orange juice, zest, honey, vinegars, and garlic. Pour dressing over salad ingredients; toss well to cover. Set aside to marinate for 15 minutes.

8. Serve the salad on individual plates topped first with the salmon and then with the grated Romano cheese.

470 calories | 22g fat | 40g carbohydrates | 29g protein | 6g sugars | 3g fiber

SALMON CHOICES
As a substitute for canned salmon, poach some fresh salmon in vegetable broth and serve chilled on top of the tomato salad. If there is no salmon to be found, canned or fresh, seared tuna fish will do, or try a piece of halibut or sea bass. The beauty of this salad is that it works no matter what protein you use.

SALMON SALAD WRAP

INGREDIENTS | SERVES 2

1 (6-ounce) can wild Alaskan salmon
¼ cup minced sweet onion
¼ cup minced celery
2 tablespoons roasted peanuts
1 tablespoon mayonnaise
1 teaspoon Dijon mustard
Salt and pepper to taste
2 tortilla wraps
2 large leaves of lettuce

Vary the amounts of mayonnaise and mustard to suit your taste or substitute roasted pine nuts for the peanuts. Feel free to improvise to ensure you get just the flavors you love.

1. Open salmon and remove and discard any pieces of skin.
2. In a medium-size bowl, combine salmon, onion, celery, peanuts, mayonnaise, mustard, salt, and pepper; mix well.
3. Heat a skillet; warm 1 tortilla at a time. Remove to individual plates.
4. Divide salmon mixture; spread along one side of a tortilla.
5. Lay lettuce along length of mixture; roll up tortilla.
6. Slice wrap in half along the diagonal and serve.

390 calories | 19g fat | 30g carbohydrates | 24g protein | 3g sugars | 3g fiber

LIME GREEN TEA PUNCH

INGREDIENTS | MAKES 2 GALLONS
12 lemon decaf green-tea bags
8 dried lime tea bags
2 gallons water
16 ounces organic lime juice
1–2 teaspoons stevia powder

Begin with 1 teaspoon of stevia and add until you have the desired sweetness. Feel free to substitute your favorite sweetener of choice.

1. Remove the tea bags from their wrappings along with the string attached to the bag.
2. In a large pasta-cooking pot, bring water to a boil.
3. Turn off heat; add tea bags. Cover; allow to steep until water has cooled.
4. When cool, remove tea bags; add lime-juice concentrate and stevia powder. Stir well to dissolve sweetener.
5. Ladle into a punch bowl; add chopped fruit if desired. Serve over ice in a glass.

150 calories | 1g fat | 45g carbohydrates | 1g protein | 6g sugars | 2g fiber

---

DESERT LIME TEA
The addition of dried lime from the Arabian Desert provides an additional dose of vitamin C along with a neat citrus flavor. Traditionally harvested and dried in the hot desert sun, it combines beautifully with the crisp flavor of the green tea.

BLACK BEAN AND CHICKEN SAUSAGE STEW

INGREDIENTS | SERVES 12

½ pound dried black beans

7 cups water

3" piece kombu sea vegetable

1 onion

1 green pepper

2 carrots

1 medium sweet potato

3 cloves garlic

1 package organic chicken sausage (6 links)

¼ cup extra-virgin olive oil

2 teaspoons cumin powder

1 teaspoon sea salt

2 tablespoons kudzu root powder

You will want to make this stew to serve your guests and family, take it along to a potluck dinner, or freeze it in individual containers for future use. Otherwise, just halve the ingredients to serve six and season with salt to taste.

1. In a large saucepan or pressure cooker, cover beans with water; soak overnight. In the morning drain, return to pot, and add 7 cups of water. Add kombu to beans; bring water to boil, reduce heat, and simmer until beans are tender, about 1 hour.

2. Meanwhile, chop onion, green pepper, and carrots; peel and chop sweet potato; and mince garlic. Slice sausage links and chop into bite-size pieces.

172

3. In a large Dutch oven, heat oil; sauté onion, pepper, carrots, and garlic until almost tender. Add cumin powder to onion mixture; stir well to combine. Add chopped sausage; allow to cook another 3 minutes. Add cooked black beans and liquid to sausage mixture; stir well.

4. Stir in sea salt; bring mixture to a boil, reduce heat, cover, and simmer until vegetables are cooked and tender, about 20 minutes, stirring occasionally.

5. In a small glass or measuring cup, dissolve kudzu-root powder with a small amount of water. Slowly add to stew, stirring as you do so. It should begin to thicken immediately, so watch for level of thickness desired.

6. Cover; allow to simmer another 1–2 minutes. Remove from heat; adjust seasonings; and serve.

150 calories | 6g fat | 18g carbohydrates | 5g protein | 3g sugars | 3g fiber

METHODS OF COOKING

You can speed up the process of cooking your beans by using a pressure cooker, which would cut the time in half. On the other hand, if you do not have the time, you can use canned black beans and prepare the vegetables with a quick sauté then add all the ingredients to a slow cooker and cook on high 3 hours or 5–6 hours on low.

SPICY MUNG BEANS IN COCONUT MILK

INGREDIENTS | SERVES 8

1 cup mung beans

4 cups water

1 onion

3 cloves garlic

1 hot pepper or 1 teaspoon red pepper flakes

2" piece fresh ginger

1 tablespoon coconut oil

1 tablespoon ghee (clarified butter)

1 teaspoon curry powder

1 teaspoon garam masala (Indian spices)

2 medium tomatoes

5.5 ounces coconut milk

½ teaspoon sea salt

Mung beans are often sprouted and used in salads and to top off Asian-style stir-fries. Traditionally, they are cooked in India, similarly to this recipe, where the dish is called a moong dhal. There is no need to presoak these beans, as they cook quickly and are easy to digest.

1. Wash and sort through the beans, removing any stones or other debris. In a large saucepan or Dutch oven, bring the beans and water to a boil over medium-high heat; cover, reduce, and allow to simmer until beans become tender, about 15 minutes.

174

2. Meanwhile, chop onion; mince garlic and pepper; and peel and mince ginger.

3. Heat oil and ghee in a skillet; sauté vegetables over medium-low heat, stirring from time to time, until onions are tender, about 4 minutes. Add curry powder and garam masala; stir well. Cook until spices release their aroma, about 1–2 minutes.

4. While onion-spice mixture is cooking, chop tomatoes; place in a blender or food processor and purée until smooth and liquid.

5. Pour tomatoes into beans along with onion-spice mixture. Add a small amount of water to skillet to wash out any remaining oil or spice adhering to the bottom of the pan; add to beans. Add coconut milk and salt to taste; stir well.

6. Reduce heat to simmer; cover and cook another 30 minutes, or until beans have broken apart and flavors are well combined. (At this point, you could place the bean mixture into a heated slow cooker and cook on low for a few hours until ready to serve.)

170 calories | 8g fat | 20g carbohydrates | 7g protein | 3g sugars | 5g fiber

CLARIFIED BUTTER
Clarified butter is regular butter that has had the milk solids and water removed, leaving behind a pure, golden-yellow butterfat. Also known as drawn butter or ghee, it has a rich butter flavor with a shelf life of several months and a much higher smoke point than most oils. You can buy it ready-made in an Indian or natural-foods market.

KALE FENNEL SALAD

INGREDIENTS | SERVES 4

1 bunch fresh kale
1 bulb fresh fennel
1 teaspoon anchovy paste (or 3 anchovy fillets)
1 shallot
¼ cup extra-virgin olive oil
2 tablespoons balsamic vinegar
½ teaspoon garlic powder
1 teaspoon agave syrup
2 tablespoons mayonnaise
¼ cup toasted pumpkin seeds

Use a high-quality mayonnaise such as the Vegenaise brand found in natural-foods stores. Commercial brands are loaded with flavorings, colorings, and preservatives plus refined sugar, which you want to avoid.

1. Wash and drain kale. Run a sharp knife down length of stem to remove leaf; set aside.
2. Cover bottom of a large skillet with ½" of water; set kale into pan. Cover, bring to a boil, reduce heat, and simmer until kale is tender but still bright green.
3. While kale is cooking, slice fennel into narrow strips; set aside.
4. In a blender or using a mortar and pestle, combine anchovy, shallot, oil, vinegar, garlic, agave, and mayonnaise; mix to a dressing consistency.

5. Rinse cooked kale under cool water, drain, and press out water. Chop kale well; place in a medium-size salad bowl along with fennel.

6. Spoon dressing over salad; toss well or serve dressing on side and serve salad on individual plates.

7. Top with toasted pumpkin seeds before eating.

280 calories | 21g fat | 22g carbohydrates | 5g protein | 3g sugars | 3g fiber

A LOW-GLYCEMIC SWEETENER

Agave syrup is made from the same cactus plant that tequila is made from. It is a low-glycemic sweetener that won't spike your blood sugar. Use it in place of honey or maple syrup when sugar is called for in your recipes.

PUMPKIN SEED CORNBREAD STUFFING

INGREDIENTS | MAKES 8 CUPS

THE CORNBREAD
1 ½ cups yellow cornmeal
½ cup whole-wheat flour
1 tablespoon baking powder
1 teaspoon sea salt
3 eggs
1 ¼ cup low-fat or nondairy milk
1 tablespoon honey
¼ cup melted butter

This cornbread recipe can be used to make stuffing or served on the side warm with a pat of butter and a drizzle of honey.

1. Preheat oven to 350°F.
2. In a large bowl, sift together cornmeal, flour, baking powder, and sea salt.
3. In a separate bowl, whisk together eggs, milk, and honey.
4. Add liquid mixture to dry ingredients; stir until just combined.
5. Meanwhile, melt butter; gently stir into cornbread mixture.
6. Pour batter into a greased 8" × 12" baking dish; bake 35–40 minutes, or until center is firm and golden brown.
7. When done, remove from oven, set aside, and allow to cool before handling.

210 calories | 9g fat | 28g carbohydrates | 7g protein | 4g sugars | 3g fiber

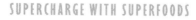

SUPERCHARGE WITH SUPERFOODS

THE STUFFING

1 pan Pumpkin Seed Cornbread (see page 178)
2 tablespoons olive oil
2 red peppers
1 medium onion
2 cloves garlic
1½ cups toasted pumpkin seeds
⅔ cup vegetable broth
1 teaspoon tamari soy sauce
½ teaspoon cayenne pepper

Complete each step of the preparation before putting the stuffing together. You can then bake it separately in the oven or stuff your turkey before baking. You can also make the stuffing a day ahead and refrigerate before baking it the next day.

1. Preheat oven to 350°F.
2. Crumble cornbread into a large bowl; set aside.
3. In a heavy skillet over medium heat, heat olive oil; sauté peppers, onion, and garlic until tender.
4. Meanwhile, in a food processor, purée pumpkin seeds, broth, tamari, and cayenne until smooth.
5. Add pumpkin-seed purée and sautéed vegetables to crumbled cornbread; mix well to combine flavors.
6. Spoon into an oiled baking dish; bake 20 minutes.

310 calories | 15g fat | 38g carbohydrates | 10g protein | 6g sugars | 4g fiber

SPICY BLENDED GREEN SALAD

INGREDIENTS

4 carrots
4 celery stalks
2 kale leaves with stem
Handful fresh parsley with stems
2 tablespoons microplant powder
1 teaspoon tamari soy sauce
Dash of hot sauce
1 teaspoon apple cider vinegar or lemon juice

1. Wash the vegetables well; chop into pieces big enough to fit into either a juicer or blender.
2. If juicing, do all the vegetables first, then stir remaining ingredients into the juice, mixing well. If blending the vegetables, add all ingredients to blender and purée until smooth.
3. Serve immediately with a celery stalk in the glass.

100 calories | 0.5g fat | 22g carbohydrates | 5g protein | 6g sugars | 6g fiber

BLENDING FRUITS
The fiber in fruits and vegetables is designed to slow down the rush of sugar to the bloodstream that can happen after eating fruit or sugar-rich carrots and beets. Blending all the vegetables with water, on the other hand, allows the nutrients and fiber to remain intact and gives you the benefits of fiber, sugar, and nutrients.

WHOLE OATS AND RAISINS

INGREDIENTS | SERVES 4

1 cup whole-oat groats
Pinch of sea salt
⅓ cup raisins
5 cups water
½ teaspoon cinnamon powder
½ cup toasted walnuts
Maple syrup to taste
Splash of milk

1. Before going to bed, combine oats, salt, raisins, water, and cinnamon in a 1.5 quart slow cooker. Turn on low; let cook overnight.
2. In the morning, chop walnuts; stir oats and spoon ½ cup into individual bowls.
3. Top with walnuts, a drizzle of maple syrup, and a splash of milk.

330 calories | 13g fat | 46g carbohydrates | 9g protein | 9g sugars | 7g fiber

WARM WINTER FOOD
Whole oats cooked slowly over a long period of time will warm your body and keep your energy levels balanced throughout the morning hours. For a more savory recipe, eliminate the raisins and cinnamon and serve with sautéed greens and toasted pumpkin seeds. Delicious either way!

SWEET-POTATO CORN CAKES WITH WASABI CREAM

INGREDIENTS | SERVES 6

1 large sweet potato
4 green onions
1 cup corn meal
⅔ cup corn kernels
1 egg
Light vegetable oil for frying
1 (10-ounce) package silken tofu
1 tablespoon plus 1 teaspoon wasabi powder
1 tablespoon ume plum vinegar
Juice of ½ lemon
Pinch of sweetener such as stevia or sugar

Silken tofu makes an excellent dairy-cream substitute for both sweet and savory recipes. The lemon juice and sweetener are used to mimic the sweet-sour taste of real cream. A finely grained salt can be substituted for the ume plum vinegar.

1. Preheat oven to 375°F. Pierce sweet-potato skin with a fork; bake until tender. Cool then peel potato.
2. Dice green onions.
3. In a large mixing bowl, combine corn meal, baked sweet potato, corn kernels, and green onions.
4. In a small bowl, whisk egg; add to cornmeal mixture.
5. Use your hands to form mixture into patties; set on a plate.

SUPERCHARGE WITH SUPERFOODS

6. Heat a small amount of oil; fry patties until brown, turning to do both sides.

7. Place on a platter and keep warm in a low-heat oven while making wasabi cream.

8. Combine tofu, wasabi powder, vinegar, lemon juice, and sweetener in a blender or food processor; purée until smooth.

9. Divide corn cakes on individual plates; top each cake with a dollop of wasabi cream.

170 calories | 2.5g fat | 30g carbohydrates | 8g protein | 3g sugars | 4g fiber

JAPANESE HORSERADISH

Wasabi is a member of the cabbage family and is cultivated in Japan. Known as Japanese horseradish, the root has a hot, strong flavor that can get your nose irritated and running if too much is eaten. Wasabi is traditionally served with sushi (raw fish), and was once used medicinally as an antidote for food poisoning.

LENTIL WALNUT PÂTÉ

INGREDIENTS | SERVES 8

½ cup walnuts

2 green onions

1½ cups cooked lentils

¾ cup cooked brown rice

3 tablespoons tamari soy sauce

¾ cup rolled oats

2 tablespoons almond butter

1. Preheat oven to 375°F.
2. Chop walnuts and green onions in food processor.
3. Combine remaining ingredients in food processor; process until smooth.
4. Spoon into a lightly oiled 8" × 8" baking pan; bake 30 minutes.
5. Cool and serve with crackers, rice cakes, or as a sandwich spread.

180 calories | 8g fat | 20g carbohydrates | 7g protein | 1g sugars | 6g fiber

WHAT TO DO WITH WALNUTS

Walnuts can be served roasted as an appetizer or coated with melted butter and honey to make a sweet, crunchy treat. Leave them raw and add them to salads, bake them in muffins and cookies, or toast them and serve over cooked grains or pasta. They can be added to stuffing (especially good with stuffed zucchinis or tomatoes) or you can chop them and add them to a baked apple or pear.

184

EASY MISO NOODLE SOUP

INGREDIENTS | SERVES 4

½ onion
2 medium carrots
2 green onions
4–6 cups vegetable broth or water
1 tablespoon dried wakame
1 cube firm tofu
4 teaspoons mellow white miso
1 (8-ounce) package cooked soba noodles
4 tablespoons toasted pumpkin seeds

*This is a delicious soup made to relax and nourish the body after a long day.
A white-colored miso will give a lighter taste than a dark-red or brown miso.
The darker the miso the longer it has fermented and the more live enzymes it will
provide. Feel free to add other vegetables or a small fillet of fish to the soup.*

1. Cut onion in thin half-moon slices; julienne carrots into matchstick shapes;
    slice green onions on diagonal into pieces.
2. Heat broth; add onion, carrot, wakame, and tofu. Simmer until onion is
    just tender.
3. Ladle broth into individual bowls; dissolve 1 teaspoon of miso into each.
4. Add ½ cup noodles to each bowl.
5. Top with pumpkin seeds and sliced green onions before serving.

180 calories | 3.5g fat | 30g carbohydrates | 10g protein | 8g sugars | 5g fiber

CARROT YOGURT SOUP

INGREDIENTS | SERVES 8

1 medium onion
1 clove garlic
4 tablespoons vegetable oil
½ teaspoon mustard seed
½ teaspoon turmeric
½ teaspoon dried ginger
½ teaspoon cumin
½ teaspoon sea salt
¼ teaspoon cayenne
¼ teaspoon cinnamon
1 pound carrots
1 tablespoon fresh lemon juice
2 cups water
2 cups low-fat plain yogurt
2 tablespoons fresh dill or 1 teaspoon dried
1 tablespoon honey
¼ teaspoon black pepper

To shorten your cooking time, consider using a pressure cooker, or if you have time to spare, follow steps 1–5 and add to a slow cooker, allowing the carrots to cook on low for 4 hours. When tender, purée the ingredients then add the yogurt, dill, honey, and pepper.

SUPERCHARGE WITH SUPERFOODS

1. Chop onion and mince garlic. In a large soup pot, sauté onion and garlic in oil until soft.
2. Add mustard seed, tumeric, ginger, cumin, sea salt, cayenne, and cinnamon. Cook for several minutes over medium heat, stirring constantly.
3. Slice carrots; add to soup pot with lemon juice and water.
4. Cover tightly; simmer until carrots are tender, about 30 minutes.
5. Purée cooked carrots and cooking liquid using a blender wand or purée in batches in a blender; return to cooking pot.
6. Add a small amount of carrot purée to yogurt, warming it slowly; whisk yogurt, dill, honey, and black pepper into carrot purée.
7. Heat mixture on low but do not boil. Ladle into soup bowls and add a fresh dollop of yogurt and a sprinkle of dill for color.

140 calories | 8g fat | 14g carbohydrates | 4g protein | 10g sugars | 2g fiber

COOKING WITH YOGURT

The beneficial bacteria in yogurt can be destroyed by high temperatures. When cooking with yogurt do not add to a boiling mixture; instead, stir the hot ingredients into the yogurt in small increments, allowing the yogurt to warm gradually. To complete, gently stir the warmed yogurt into the hot mixture.

APPENDIX A:
GLOSSARY

Allicin
A sulfur element found in garlic and known for its ability to cleanse and purify the body.

Anthocyanins
Any of various soluble glycoside pigments producing blue-to-red coloring in flowers and plants.

Antioxidants
Any of various substances (beta-carotene, vitamin C, and alpha-tocopherol) that inhibit oxidation or reactions promoted by oxygen and peroxides and help protect the body from free-radical damage.

Beano
A particular enzyme product that helps digest the carbohydrates that feed intestinal bacteria-causing gas in the intestines.

189

Beta-carotene
A member of the carotenoids, highly pigmented fat-soluble compounds naturally present in many fruits, grains, oils, and vegetables that can be converted to active vitamin A.

Beta-glucans
Polysaccharides that occur in the outer layer or bran of cereal grains.

Beta-sitosterol
The plant equivalent of cholesterol in animals, found in avocados; helps lower the amounts of cholesterol in the bloodstream.

Bioflavonoids
A group of naturally occurring plant compounds that act primarily as plant pigments and antioxidants.

Caffeic acid
A naturally occurring compound shown to be a carcinogenic inhibitor.

Catechins
A type of flavonoid and strong antioxidant that combats harmful free radicals and protects DNA.

Chitinases
A substance in avocados, bananas, and chestnuts associated with latex-fruit syndrome.

Chlorophyll

A molecule specifically designed to absorb sunlight and use this energy to synthesize carbohydrates from CO_2 and water.

Collagen

The most abundant protein in the body; needed to form bone, cartilage, skin, and tendons.

Cruciferous vegetables

A family of vegetables that includes kale, collards, Brussels sprouts, broccoli, and cauliflower; high in cancer-fighting sulforaphane compounds.

Diuretic

Foods or herbs that help dispel fluids from the body.

Enzymes

Proteins that speed up chemical reactions in the body such as the breakdown and assimilation of food in the digestive system.

Epicatechin

A group of chemicals called flavonols, shown to improve cardiovascular function and increase blood flow to the brain.

Essential fatty acids

Omega-3 and omega-6; these are essential fats needed by the body to protect against inflammation and other factors.

Ferulic acid
A potent antioxidant that is able to scavenge free radicals and protect against oxidative damage.

Flavonoids
Known for their antioxidant activity, they can help prevent free-radical damage to the body's cells. This results in protection against cancer and heart disease.

Folate
The natural form of folic acid; known as vitamin B9, and required for DNA synthesis and cell growth. It is important for red blood cell formation and energy production as well as the forming of amino acids.

Free radical
Specially reactive atom or group of atoms that has one or more unpaired electrons, produced in the body by natural biological processes or introduced from outside (tobacco smoke, toxins, or pollutants). Can damage cells, proteins, and DNA by altering their chemical structure.

Glucosinolate
A phytonutrient that actually boosts your body's detoxification enzymes, clearing potentially carcinogenic substances more quickly from your body.

Indole-3-carbinol

A compound that helps deactivate a potent estrogen metabolite (4-hydroxyestrone) that promotes tumor growth; shown to suppress not only breast-tumor cell growth but also the movement of cancerous cells to other parts of the body.

Lactobacillus acidophilus

One of the most important friendly intestinal bacteria (microflora) and necessary for gastrointestinal health.

Lutein and zeaxanthin

Compounds called xanthophylls or carotenoids related to beta-carotene. They give vegetables like carrots their orange color and add yellow pigment to plants. They are also found in large amounts in the lens and retina of the eye, where they function as antioxidants to protect the eyes from free-radical damage.

Lycopene

An antioxidant and open-chain unsaturated carotenoid that gives the red color to tomatoes and other fruits.

Lysine

An amino acid essential for tissue growth and repair.

Macronutrients

Include carbohydrates, fats, and proteins. These are the foods the body uses for energy and growth.

Micronutrients
Include vitamins and minerals.

Moles
A form of measurement of the actual number of atoms or molecules in an object.

Monounsaturated fats
Containing one double or triple bond per molecule. Canola and olive oils are rich in monounsaturated fatty acids.

Nucleic acids
RNA/DNA responsible for the renewal, repair, and growth of the cells.

Oleic acid
A form of monounsaturated fat found in avocado and shown to help lower cholesterol in the body.

Phenylethylamine
A strong stimulant related to the amphetamine family known to increase the activity of neurotransmitters in parts of the brain that control your ability to pay attention and stay alert.

Phytic acid
Present in the bran and hulls of all seeds; it can block the uptake of essential minerals in the digestive tract.

SUPERCHARGE WITH SUPERFOODS

Phytonutrients
Antioxidants that disarm free radicals before they can damage DNA, cell membranes, and fat-containing molecules such as cholesterol.

Phytosterol
Plant sterols structurally similar to cholesterol that act in the intestine to lower cholesterol absorption.

Polyphenols
An antioxidant phytochemical that tends to prevent or neutralize the damaging effects of free radicals.

Polyunsaturated fats
Having in each molecule many chemical bonds, in which two or three pairs of electrons are shared by two atoms.

Probiotics
Beneficial microflora (good bacteria) found in the intestines.

Quercetin
A yellow crystalline pigment, usually occurring in the form of glycosides, in various plants; proven to prevent unstable oxygen molecules or free radicals from damaging cells.

Saponins
A bitter substance found in plants' seed coats that repels birds and insects.

Saturated fats
Animal and dairy fats that remain solid at room temperature.

Sofrito
A method of adding sautéed onions, garlic, herbs, and spices to enhance a soup or bean dish.

Sulforaphane
A phytonutrient compound found in broccoli shown to prevent the development of tumors.

Theanine
An amino acid present in the tea plant. Absorbed by the small intestine, it crosses the blood-brain barrier, where it affects the brain's neurotransmitters and increases alpha brain-wave activity.

Theobromine
A caffeine-like substance found in chocolate; when taken in excess can inhibit the body's ability to absorb minerals.

SUPERCHARGE WITH SUPERFOODS

APPENDIX B:
RESOURCE GUIDE

NATURAL FOOD SUPPLIES

Nature's Harvest
P.O. Box 291, 28 Main Street, Blairstown, NJ 07825
Contact Michelle St. Andre: 908-362-6766
Harvest6766@embarqmail.com

Organic Produce
www.diamondorganics.com

Whole Grains and Sea Vegetables
www.kushistore.com/acatalog/welcome.html

Organic Foods and Products
www.diamondorganics.com

Earthbound Farm, Vegetables
www.ebfarm.com

Cascadian Farms, Frozen Fruits and Vegetables
www.cfarm.com

Seeds of Change, Organic Tomato Sauces and Salsas
www.seedsofchange.com

Green Mountain Coffee Roasters (Organic, Sustainably Grown, Fair Trade)
www.greenmountaincoffee.com

HEALTH-EDUCATION WEBSITES

Dr. Joseph Mercola
www.mercola.com

Organic Consumers Association
www.organicconsumers.org

ENERGY-CONSUMPTION STATISTICS

Energy Information Administration Website
www.eia.doe.gov/kids/classactivities/CrunchTheNumbersIntermediateDec2002.pdf

Saving with Recycling, NRDC Website

www.nrdc.org/land/forests/gtissue.asp

Saving with Compact Fluorescents, Environmental Defense Website

www.environmentaldefense.org/article.cfm?contentid=5215

SUSTAINABLE BUILDING AND RETROFITTING

Bob Swain's Website

www.bobswain.com

General Building Information

www.greenbuilder.com

Alternative Energy Systems, Products, and Installation

www.utilityfree.com

Saline Pool Systems

www.salinepoolsystems.com

Sick Building Syndrome

www.wellbuilding.com

RENEWABLE RESOURCES

www.green-e.org

www.greenfacts.org

OTHER RESOURCES

Cleaning Chemicals
www.restoreproducts.com

Tom Foerstel's Website for Organic Products
www.organic.org
www.organiclinks.com

Daliya Robson's Website for Nontoxic Household Furnishings
www.nontoxic.com

For Sustainably Harvested Household Products
www.seventhgeneration.com

Chemical-Free Home Products
www.EnvironProducts.com

Measuring Your Environmental Footprint
www.carbonfootprint.com

What the Labels Really Say
www.truthinlabeling.org

INDEX

SUPERCHARGE WITH SUPERFOODS